THE OFFICIAL
GOLD'S GYM
BEGINNER'S GUIDE TO FITNESS

THE AUTHORITY ON FITNESS SINCE 1965

DAVID PORTER

McGraw·Hill

New York   Chicago   San Francisco   Lisbon   London   Madrid   Mexico City
Milan   New Delhi   San Juan   Seoul   Singapore   Sydney   Toronto

Library of Congress Cataloging-in-Publication Data

Porter, David, 1960–
    The Official Gold's Gym beginner's guide to fitness / by David Porter.
      p.   cm.
    Includes index.
    ISBN 0-07-142282-X

    1. Physical fitness. 2. Exercise. I. Title: Beginner's guide to
    fitness. II. Gold's Gym. III. Title.

  GV481.P59 2005
  613.7—dc22   2004008275

1 2 3 4 5 6 7 8 9 0   QPD/QPD   3 2 1 0 9 8 7 6 5 4

ISBN 0-07-142282-X

McGraw-Hill books are available at special quantity discounts to use as premiums and sales promotions, or for use in corporate training programs. For more information, please write to the Director of Special Sales, Professional Publishing, McGraw-Hill, Two Penn Plaza, New York, NY 10121-2298. Or contact your local bookstore.

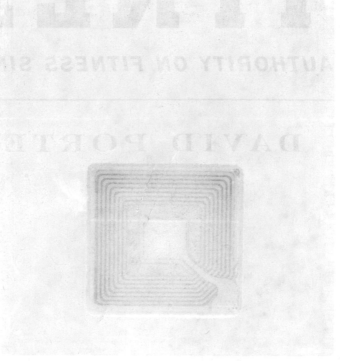

This book is printed on acid-free paper.

CONTENTS

ACKNOWLEDGMENTS

This book was developed and produced by Mountain Lion, Inc., a book producer specializing in fitness, sports, and general reference books. A book producer relies on the special skills of many people. The following contributed to producing this book; to all of them we say "thanks."

- Mark Weinstein, editor at McGraw-Hill Trade, whose guidance and suggestions were instrumental in moving this project through its various stages
- Ed Powderly, Senior Vice President of Product Licensing of Gold's Gym International, who contributed significantly to formulating the book's overall content, including the editorial scope and photographic treatment
- Maureen Babcock of Gold's Gym, who gathered and sent us the appropriate Gold's Gym apparel for our fitness demonstrators
- Ken Strickland, former U.S. Marine Corps Sergeant Major and manager of the Gold's Gym located on the outskirts of Princeton, New Jersey, who arranged and coordinated our photography sessions (Ken runs his gym facility with an exemplary *esprit de corps,* pursuing his fitness mission with an infectious enthusiasm.)

- Randy and Bonnie Vey, owners and operators of the spectacular and award-winning Princeton Gold's Gym facility, and their staff
- John Monteleone and Vicki Russo at Mountain Lion, Inc., who shepherded the project from concept to finished manuscript and completed photographs
- David Porter, who researched and wrote the text
- Tracy Carroll of The Anatomical Edge (Houston, Tex.) and Gerard K. Green, strength and conditioning coach for the Rider University (Lawrenceville, N.J.) athletic teams, for their contributions to the men's and women's beginner and intermediate programs
- Jeanie Subach, M.A., R.D., L.D.N., nutrition consultant for the Philadelphia Eagles and Philadelphia 76ers, for her contributions to the section on nutrition for athletes
- The Association of Professional Team Physicians, for information on stretching and strengthening exercises and injury prevention
- Barry Havens, photographer, who expertly handled all the photography
- Debby Bocchino, Paul Coldren, and Kim Kasics, our Gold's Stars, who ably demonstrated the exercises in all of the beginner workout programs

INTRODUCTION

We live in a country of paradoxes, particularly when it comes to health and physical well-being. We are obsessed with fitness, yet we rank near the top in the percentage of our population that is obese. We are slaves to all manner of high-tech gadgets that are supposed to free up more time for us to improve our personal lives and be more active, yet ours is one of the most sedentary cultures in the world.

Along with the faster pace of life and the stresses it produces, we are bombarded with images that tell us what we should look like, from the sculpted male physiques on the covers of glossy magazines to the rail-thin actresses starring in the latest summer blockbusters. At the same time, we are bombarded with television commercials hyping products and programs that promise to turn our flab into rock-hard muscle in just minutes a day.

The reality, of course, is different. It is a fine goal to want six-pack abs, but it is a more realistic and rewarding goal to want to increase your cardiovascular capacity or your muscle strength and endurance. If the sculpted abs come along with it, so much the better.

Even if exercise and getting in good physical shape didn't make you look better and feel better about yourself, it would still be well worth the time and effort. Many of the benefits of regular exercise are obvious, but some are not. Perhaps more important is what may happen to you if you don't exercise regularly.

A recent publication by the President's Council on Physical Fitness and Sports reported the following facts:

- A moderate amount of physical activity—as little as 15 to 30 minutes of walking, running, or even raking leaves per day—can yield significant health benefits. These benefits only increase with greater amounts of activity.
- Moderate daily physical activity can reduce the risk of cardiovascular disease, type-2 diabetes, and certain types of cancer. It can also lower blood pressure and cholesterol levels, prevent or slow the development of osteoporosis, and help reduce obesity and symptoms of anxiety, depression, and arthritis.
- A sedentary lifestyle is a major risk factor in a variety of preventable diseases: Forty percent of deaths in the U.S. are caused by behavior patterns that could be modified.
- Up to 300,000 preventable deaths per year in the United States can be attributed in part to physical inactivity.
- Four in 10 American adults say that they are not physically active at all, and seven in 10 report that they don't engage in the recommended amount of moderate exercise on a daily or weekly basis.

- Physically inactive people are twice as likely to develop coronary disease as people who are regularly active.
- The health risks posed by physical inactivity are almost as high as the risks created by cigarette smoking, high blood pressure, and high cholesterol.
- Inactivity combined with a poor diet can lead to obesity, and people who are obese are at increased risk for high blood pressure, diabetes, coronary heart disease, stroke, gall bladder disease, osteoarthritis, sleep apnea, respiratory problems, and certain types of cancer.
- Sixty-one percent of American adults were obese in a study conducted in 1999. In direct and indirect medical costs, obesity costs more than $100 billion annually.
- The main obstacles for most people who need to increase their level of physical activity are time, access to facilities, and safe environments for exercise.

The last point is particularly important. People know that they *should* exercise; creating the time in their schedules to actually do it on a regular basis is the true challenge. This issue is addressed in this book, along with tips on how to stay motivated and stick with your exercise program once you've started.

As the title implies, *The Official Gold's Gym Beginner's Guide to Fitness* is for adults who want to improve their personal fitness but may be unfamiliar with fitness training. You may be in your twenties and have never lifted weights or run on a treadmill. You may be a former high school athlete, now in your thirties, who hasn't worked out in 15 years but wants to get back in shape again. You may be a 35-year-old woman who wants to stay in shape while she's pregnant. Or you may be in your mid-forties and want to im-

prove your performance in a particular sport.

Your specific goals will surely be different from those of the person on the treadmill next to you at the gym. Like you, the people in all of the scenarios above require a basic understanding of what goes into physical fitness, as well as the ability to put that knowledge into practice.

The Official Gold's Gym Beginner's Guide to Fitness gives you the tools to become physically fit; it is up to you to make fitness a reality.

An old friend of mine, who didn't play organized sports in high school or college, hardly fit the profile of an athlete. He became interested in distance running in his late twenties, however, and gradually worked his way up to competing in marathons. Eventually, he could run the 26 miles in 2 hours, 45 minutes. (He would have placed 150th in the field of more than 30,000 runners in the 2002 New York City Marathon.) The moral of the story: You never know what your limits are until you test them.

The Official Gold's Gym Beginner's Guide to Fitness won't turn you into the next Lance Armstrong or help you win bodybuilding contests. It *will* help you improve your fitness level, which in turn will improve your health. It *will* help you replace fat with muscle, increase your strength and energy, improve balance and flexibility, and reverse bone loss.

This book features tips on getting started and staying motivated, warming up and stretching, choosing the right exercises for your specific goals, avoiding injuries, and eating the right food.

Also included are descriptions and photographs of the latest weight exercises for your upper and lower back, chest, shoulders, arms, abdominals and torso, buttocks, and legs. Instructors with years of experience in personal training offer their own tips, as well as basic workout programs for men and women, starting with beginner-level exercises and gradually working up to more intense workouts. Personal accounts of individual club members describe why they began working out, how they achieved success in the gym, and how it has improved their lifestyle.

While this book concentrates primarily on weight training, it also includes valuable information on different types of aerobic conditioning, flexibility training, and even alternative training—which can help you maintain your workout schedule and fitness level when you can't get to the gym.

The Official Gold's Gym Beginner's Guide to Fitness is a comprehensive source of information for anyone who wants to reap the benefits of improved fitness. Use this book as a starting point for creating your own fitness story.

1

Getting Started

You have decided to start a physical fitness program. This takes a serious commitment from you—a mental, emotional, and time commitment. Starting and stopping a program will do little good. You must believe in the benefits of fitness, because that will keep you motivated and committed to the program you select.

The mental aspect is important. You can't regain in a few days or weeks what you may have lost during years of sedentary living, but you can experience progress and good fitness if you stick with a program. You'll need to set your mind to it and have the same kind of willpower that a dieter needs to be successful.

There is a prize to be won down the road. Go for the prize.

As you undertake your fitness program, it is important to remember that fitness is an individual quality that varies from person to person. It is influenced by age, sex, heredity, personal habits, exercise, and eating practices. You can't do anything about the first three factors. But it *is* within your power to make changes in the other three.

GETTING A CHECKUP

According to the President's Council on Physical Fitness and Sports, if you are under 35 and in good health, you probably don't need to see a doctor before beginning an exercise program. But if you are over 35 and/or have been inactive for several years, you should consult your physician, who may recommend a graded exercise test.

You need to see a doctor first if any of the following conditions apply to you.

- High blood pressure
- Heart trouble
- A family history of early stroke or heart attack deaths
- Frequent dizzy spells
- Extreme breathlessness after mild exertion
- Arthritis or other bone problems
- Severe muscle, ligament, or tendon problems
- A known or suspected disease

Vigorous exercise creates minimal health risks for persons in good health or who are following a doctor's advice.

Much greater risks are taken by those who are habitually inactive and obese.

If you are still unsure as to whether you should see a doctor before starting a fitness program, the President's Council recommends that you answer the following questions.

- Has a doctor ever told you that you have heart trouble?
- Do you suffer frequently from chest pains?
- Do you often feel faint or have spells of severe dizziness?
- Has a doctor ever told you that your blood pressure is too high?
- Has a doctor ever told you that you have a bone or joint problem, such as arthritis, that has been or could be aggravated by exercise?
- Are you over the age of 65 and not accustomed to exercise?
- Are you taking prescription medications, such as those that treat high blood pressure?
- Is there a good medical reason why you should not begin an exercise program?

If you answered "yes" to any of these questions, you should consult your doctor *before* beginning an exercise program.

WHAT TO WEAR

Walk into almost any sporting goods store, and the clothing and accessories department will make you dizzy. From the vast array of fashionable workout clothing, you should select clothing that is comfortable, safe, and suitable for the conditions in which you'll be exercising.

If you will be exercising outdoors, do you live in a warm or cold climate? What season is it?

What form of exercise will you be undertaking? (Baggy clothes can be dangerous on exercise equipment, and tight-fitting clothes can restrict your movement on a basketball or tennis court.)

How long will your workouts last, and how intensely will you exert yourself?

Weather Conditions

Unless you plan to exercise only in a gym, the weather will dictate what you wear for exercising. There are several important points to keep in mind so that you are comfortable at any temperature and are able to get the most out of your workout.

In warm weather, you need to let your body breathe so that it can cool itself by sweating when you exercise. Otherwise, you risk heat exhaustion or, in extreme cases, heat stroke.

Light-colored, cotton clothing is the best to wear in warm weather. Never wear rubberized or plastic clothing, since these materials can cause your body temperature to rise dramatically. A hat can keep the sun off your face, and it can be soaked in cold water to keep your head cool.

In cold weather, you need to trap your body heat. Wear layers of clothing, with cotton as the first layer. The clothes shouldn't be bulky, since that will restrict movement. If you get too warm, you can shed a layer, but be careful not to shed too much, because your sweat may cool quickly if you do. A light windbreaker worn on top of other layers of clothing can protect you against both wind and cold. To avoid the risk of hypothermia in extremely cold weather, exposed skin should be kept at a minimum. A wool hat can also help you retain body heat.

What to Wear for Exercise

Exercise clothing should be loose enough to permit freedom of movement and should make you feel comfortable and self-assured. Comfortable clothes should not bind or restrict your movement. Watch out for seams and likely chafing areas, particularly on the insides of the thighs.

As a general rule, since exercise generates a large amount of body heat, you should wear less clothing than you would if you weren't exercising. Light-colored clothing that reflects the sun's rays is cooler in the summer, and dark clothing is warmer in the winter.

What to Wear for Weight Training

When you are training with weights, you should generally wear what you would wear when you are playing a sport or doing other exercises. However, there are some specific guidelines and gear that can enhance your weight training program.

Clothing

Your normal exercise wear will usually suffice unless you need more support for your muscles and joints, in which case you may want to wear clothing that is made of expandable material. Clothes that fit more snugly also allow you to see whether your body is angled correctly and you are doing the exercises properly. Don't wear baggy tops or bottoms that can get caught in weights or exercise machines.

Shoes

Always wear shoes when you are in a weight room; this helps prevent injury in case you or someone else drops a weight on your foot. Special weight-lifting shoes manufactured by major shoe manufacturers give you good balance and support, but you can use any type of cross-training shoe that offers lateral support. Running shoes should be avoided, because their wider and raised soles can cause your ankle to roll to the outside.

Gloves

Specially designed weightlifting gloves can protect your hands from chafing and callusing, which can result from continuous grasping of barbells and dumbbells. Ask your coach or trainer for a recommendation.

Belts

Weightlifting belts are used by competitive power lifters, but they can be useful for athletes at all levels. They help support your abdominal muscles and lower back when you are lifting heavy weights, particularly when you are doing exercises like squats, hex bar dead lifts, and Olympic-style exercises. These belts are not necessary for exercises that do not place stress on your back. Check with your coach or trainer about using a weightlifting belt—but remember that proper technique is the best safeguard against injury.

Braces and Supports

Braces and supports are used most often to allow athletes to continue to train while recovering from a joint or muscle injury. Braces, which frequently feature hard plastic or metal hinges, restrict range of motion and are typically used after an acute injury. Supports, which consist of padding, wraps, or other soft materials, allow greater range of motion and help compress the affected area and keep it warm. However, supports can cause discomfort and even injury if they are too tight. Always consult your physician or orthopedist before attempting to return to weight training after an injury.

Athletic Shoes

Athletic shoes have changed dramatically over the years, to the point that you can choose a pair of shoes designed specifically for almost every activity. All those choices, however, can make buying shoes more confusing than ever. Aside from cost, there's little excuse for not selecting the proper footwear.

Here are some general tips for purchasing athletic shoes:

- If you think that you need new athletic shoes, you probably do. Athletic shoes don't last forever, and many injuries can be prevented by replacing old, worn-out shoes with new ones.
- When shopping for athletic shoes, wear the same socks you will be wearing while exercising. Also, try on shoes later in the day, when your feet have expanded. This will help you get a more accurate fit, since your foot can increase as much as half a size while you are exercising.
- Base your purchasing decision on fit and comfort, not on brand reputation. With a plethora of shoe manufacturers on the market, you should try out more than one or two brands, unless you have gotten good results in the past and want to stay with one brand.
- Aim for a little more width in the front of the shoe and a little less in the back. Your toes should have plenty of room, but your heel should be prevented from moving around too much inside the shoe. Otherwise, you risk forming blisters. In the heel, too much cushioning can cause Achilles tendinitis.

Cross-Training Shoes

Cross-training shoes are hybrids, in a sense. They have a thicker sole than a tennis shoe, but not as thick as a running shoe. They are built with enough cushioning and shock absorption to run several miles on a roadway, but they also have enough lateral support to allow you to play tennis or basketball without the risk of turning your ankle.

Despite their versatility, cross-training shoes are not the be-all and end-all of athletic footwear. The key point is to buy shoes that fit your needs. If you will spend a significant amount of time walking, jogging, or running on the treadmill or roadway, you should buy running shoes to minimize the risk of foot, ankle, knee, and back problems in the near future. For lifting weights or playing basketball or tennis or other sports, you may want to buy cross-training shoes.

Women's Footwear

Women's feet are different from men's, a fact that took the athletic shoe industry some time to realize. Fortunately, manufacturers are now more in tune with the specific needs of women athletes and have designed shoes accordingly. This often means that women's shoes have additional arch support to lessen pronation (the rotation of the feet inward), thereby decreasing the risk of knee inflammation or injury.

Sports Bras

The best sports bras are designed to provide support without discomfort caused by friction. As in choosing athletic shoes, you should try on several different types of sports bras to determine which is best for your activity level and type.

Sports bras come in two basic styles: compression bras, which don't use cups but bring your breasts closer to your rib cage by compressing them, and encapsulation bras, which use cups and usually have some form of underwire support. Encapsulation bras offer greater support for large-breasted women, but typically have straps and other features that can cause chafing.

To get the right fit, make sure that the bra gives you freedom of movement in your upper body while minimizing chest bouncing. It shouldn't be so tight that it hinders your breathing during exertion, when you will need your full lung capacity.

Here are some general tips for purchasing a sports bra:

- Keep in mind the activity or activities you will be performing. High-impact activities like running and basketball require more support than walking or cross-country skiing.
- Choose a sports bra that fits right, even if it is not the same size as your regular bra. When trying on a bra in the store, try to simulate the movements you will be performing during exercise.
- As with athletic shoes, sports bras gradually lose their elasticity and wear out. Depending on how frequently you exercise, you may need to replace a sports bra every six months to a year.
- Smooth, seamless cups can prevent bruising and irritation.
- Look for a snug fit: the more your breasts move, the greater risk there is of chafing and irritation.
- Look for bras that have clasps, tags, and straps covered by fabric so that they don't dig into your skin.
- Avoid nylon stitching.
- Choose models with wide shoulder straps, since these are less likely to cut into your shoulders than thin straps.

2

Making Time
and Staying Motivated

"I'd get in shape, but I don't have the time. . . ."

How often have you heard that line (or said it yourself)?

Guess what! Everyone is busy—that's the way life is. But busy people can make time for staying in good physical shape. This chapter offers tips for making time and staying motivated, plus some testimonials from real people who make it happen every day, every week, every month.

Schedule your workout as if it were a business appointment that you cannot miss. If you *schedule* your normal workout time in the morning, you won't be inclined to think, "Oh, I can go later." Later becomes never, and often very quickly.

Keep a workout log, described in Chapter 8. This keeps you honest. It provides physical proof for the number of workouts you have actually done in a week. It prevents you from deluding yourself into thinking that you went to the gym last Monday, when actually you went out for coffee instead.

Repeat to yourself that this activity is *for you.* You are not doing this for anyone else, except indirectly or in the long run, perhaps. You are paying yourself—just like your job pays you—only the payment is in the form of better health and an increased energy level. You may also be paid in lower medical costs and less missed work; people who exercise regularly miss less work and are more productive than those who don't.

The people who have the hardest time getting to the gym or exercising at home are parents of children under the age of 12. If you are in this category, consider exercising with your kids. Buy a bike seat for your kid or a carrier to attach to your bike. Find a way to incorporate the family into an exercise routine. Even if you only manage 15 minutes of exercise at a time, it quickly adds up if you do it regularly.

Morning is the most productive time of day for many people, and this can be vital to developing good workout habits. Getting up early and working out before you go to work gets

GOLD'S STARS

Avery, 37, personal trainer/nutritionist

Avery got an early start in fitness through her parents, who involved her in activities like running and aerobics. She's carried over that philosophy by trying to include others in her workout activities. She began exercising seriously in the mid-1980s after a friend got her interested, and she has been able to maintain a good level of fitness ever since. She understands that a workout partner waiting for you at the gym on a certain day is a strong motivational tool—you don't want to let them down.

Like most people who work out regularly, Avery has gone through periods where she has hit a plateau in her training. At those times, she finds it helpful to get away from the gym for a little while and explore other activities. "I usually find something I like to do, like walking, riding a bike, or yoga," she says. "I like to be physical."

For the times when she has lost a little conditioning from taking time off, Avery says that she reminds herself to lift less weight than she was lifting when she left off.

Other than that, she says, it's pretty easy to get back into a comfortable routine.

Mike, 27, landscaper

The toughest time to make it to the gym is after a long day at work, says Mike, who has been a bodybuilder since he was 19. Even if he feels worn out, he reminds himself that this is something he enjoys and is doing for himself. If his workouts get stale or he hits a plateau, Mike takes the initiative and changes his workouts, tinkering with different exercises and different numbers of sets and repetitions.

For beginners, Mike recommends using lighter weights and higher repetitions, which has the dual effect of getting you used to the lifting motion and cutting down on the risk of injury. "As you get used to it," he says, "you can progress, little by little."

Even though looking at Mike's physique could make almost anybody feel intimidated, he says the key to a successful workout is to focus directly and exclusively on your own routine.

"You can't look at everybody else," he says. "You've got to do what you can do."

Angela, 44, writer/editor

Exchanging an unhealthy habit for a healthy one brought Angela to the gym nine years ago, and she hasn't looked back. She had decided to quit smoking, but needed an outlet for her excess energy and tension, so she joined a gym and began running on the treadmill. She eventually started lifting weights too.

Angela found that she was very competitive and would play little games with herself as she was working out, which had the effect of making her push herself harder. She also discovered that there was a social component in going to the gym, and she has made friends with some of the other regulars.

With a full-time job and a family now, she finds it difficult to work out at the same time every week, but she manages to get in her three or four days anyway.

"It has to be one of the things that you're *going* to do," Angela says. "If I haven't gone for a couple of days, it goes to the top of the list for the next day. It's not that I feel I *have* to do it; it's that I know I'll feel better when I do it."

you energized for the day (assuming you got enough sleep the night before, of course). It also ensures that your workout doesn't get crowded out by something that crops up later in the day, and it saves you from having to fit the gym into a busy day of meetings. The genuine physical bonus is elevating your metabolic rate the very first thing in the day. You are ahead of the game, rather than trying to play catch-up on all the food you have eaten that day.

Here are some more tips to keep you going in your workout schedule:

- Choose activities you enjoy, whether they involve going to the gym or exercising outdoors.
- Set realistic goals and reward yourself when you achieve them.
- Adopt a specific fitness plan and write it down.
- Keep a log to record your progress. Include your weight and other relevant statistics.
- Upgrade your fitness program as you progress. Keep challenging yourself.
- Vary your activities.
- Avoid injuries by pacing yourself and by including a warm-up and

a cooldown period as part of every workout. There's nothing worse than being injured and having to cut back on your activities.

- Enlist the support and encourage the participation of your family and friends.

- Enlist another person to be an exercise partner. This can have great benefits for both of you.
- Associate with people who share your views about the importance of physical fitness.

3

Types of Training

You've decided to start an exercise program and improve your physical fitness—that's the first step. Now what? Do you join your neighborhood Gold's Gym? Go out and buy expensive home exercise equipment? Call an 800 number you saw on TV and order the latest gadgets that promise to give you a cut physique in five minutes per day or less?

The next step is to decide what goal(s) you want to pursue:

- Increasing muscle strength
- Increasing muscle endurance
- Increasing flexibility
- Increasing cardiorespiratory endurance
- Losing weight

You probably want to achieve a combination of these goals, since they are interrelated anyway. First, though, let's focus on the last goal in the list, losing weight.

GETTING FIT VS. LOSING WEIGHT

This may seem an odd concept. Getting fit *means* losing weight, doesn't it?

Well, as those rental car commercials like to repeat . . . not exactly.

As you follow the programs described later in this book or come up with your own, you may find that you are not actually losing weight. If this is the case, don't panic—you're probably healthier than you think. Studies have shown that people who are a little overweight but in good physical shape are healthier than people who are not overweight but not in shape.

This means that the person in the next cubicle at the office who skips lunch two days a week and just nibbles at his/her food the rest of the time may fit into smaller clothes sizes than you, but is not necessarily healthier—especially if you are exercising and he or she is not. Just because you may not achieve your "ideal weight" right away—or ever, perhaps—does not mean that your exercise program is not providing you with tangible benefits like lower cholesterol levels, lower blood pressure, and increased cardiovascular efficiency. Keep in mind, too, that muscle weighs more than fat.

The relationship between exercising and losing weight will be addressed in more detail in Chapter 11 on nutrition. The best way to lose weight is to combine exercise with a decrease in the amount of calories you consume each day.

We all know that consuming fewer calories is easier said than done, especially since people who are more active need more energy than people who are sedentary. But it doesn't have to be a Herculean chore. For instance, if you take 15 minutes to walk a mile, you'll burn about 100 extra calories. If you walk a mile every day, this amounts to 700 extra calories a week and about 35,000 calories a year! That's equivalent to losing 10 pounds, since each pound of fat your body stores represents 3,500 calories of unused energy.

On the flip side, you can easily add 10 pounds in a year just by eating 100 extra calories a day without increasing your level of physical activity. An extra slice of bread or an extra soft drink a day is all it takes. To gain weight that is lean muscle mass and not extra fat, however, you need to increase the number of calories you consume at the same time you are exercising regularly.

COMPONENTS OF FITNESS

There are four basic components of fitness: cardiorespiratory endurance, muscle strength, muscle endurance, and flexibility. Since these terms appear throughout this book, let's define them:

- **Cardiorespiratory endurance:** The ability to deliver oxygen and nutrients to tissues, and to remove wastes, over sustained periods of time. Long runs and swims are among the methods employed in measuring this component. Can your heart and lungs function efficiently over a sustained period? When you are fit, they easily deliver

oxygen and nutrients to tissues and remove wastes.
- **Muscle strength:** The ability of a muscle to exert force for a brief period of time. Upper-body strength, for example, can be measured by various weightlifting exercises. Are you able to lift a variety of weights easily? When your muscles are fit, they can exert force for a burst of activity.
- **Muscle endurance:** The ability of a muscle, or a group of muscles, to sustain repeated contractions or to continue applying force against a fixed object. Push-ups are often used to test the endurance of arm and shoulder muscles. When you are fit, your muscles can exert force over a sustained period of time.
- **Flexibility:** The ability to move joints and use muscles through their full range of motion.

TYPES OF EXERCISE

There are four basic types of exercise: aerobic, stretching, strengthening, and anaerobic. As the specific programs outlined later in this book describe, your weekly exercise routine should include some of each type of exercise, even though you won't be doing each type in every workout.

You should begin and end all workouts with stretching to improve flexibility and avoid injury, but you should pursue aerobic activities (for example, jogging and swimming) and anaerobic activities (for example, weight lifting) on alternate days. The key is to pick the right activities that develop and maintain each of the basic components of fitness—and help you meet your specific goals at the same time.

Aerobic Exercise: The Basis

Aerobic exercise is the basic building block of any fitness program. It strengthens your heart, increases your ability to use oxygen, releases stress, and burns fat and calories. The more often you exercise aerobically, the more benefit to your body (within reason, of course; pushing yourself too much can result in overtraining, a phenomenon discussed later in this book).

The word *aerobic* comes from two Greek words meaning "oxygen" and "life." All physical movement requires energy (calories)—believe it or not, you can burn 90 calories an hour when you're sleeping—but the type of exercise that uses the most energy is aerobic exercise. Any activity that you perform in a continuous, rhythmic movement and that uses your body's large muscle groups can be considered an aerobic exercise. Jogging, brisk walking, swimming, biking, cross-country skiing, and aerobic dancing are some of the more popular forms of aerobic activities.

Regular aerobic exercise will improve the ability of your heart, lungs, blood vessels, and tissues to use oxygen to produce energy.

Stretching and Flexibility: Priming the Parts

The benefits of stretching are obvious, but they bear repeating. Stretching is one of the best ways to prevent injury and soreness. It gets the blood flowing to your muscles and prepares them for the stresses you are going to place on them during your workout. After you are finished exercising, it cools your muscles down and prevents tightening and soreness.

In general, stretching helps you increase your range of motion so that not only will you be protecting yourself from injury, but you will find it easier to perform many of the movements required in an exercise program or specific sport.

Chapter 6 is devoted to specific types of stretches for all areas of the body. Anyone who has suffered an injury as a result of muscles that were too tight will tell you that, for the amount of time it takes to do it, stretching more than repays the effort you put into it.

Strengthening

There are many kinds of strengthening exercises, but the most common use weights to provide resistance. Weight training is an example of an anaerobic activity (short bursts of activity at near-maximum intensity). During weight training, you will often find that you are not working up a sweat. You are burning fewer calories than you do during aerobic exercise, when you are moving constantly. But the benefits of weight training are numerous:

- Weight training builds muscle, and this muscle increases the rate at which you burn calories throughout the day, since muscle needs more calories than fat.
- Muscle weighs more than fat, so you may look and feel thinner even though your weight remains the same (and you'll certainly be healthier).
- Dieting causes you to lose muscle as well as fat. Weight training helps you build that muscle back up, which can result in a leaner, healthier body.
- Resistance exercises may help prevent osteoporosis, a loss of bone density that usually occurs in older people.

Anaerobic Exercise

Anaerobic exercise involves short bursts of activity at a maximum or near-maximum level of output. Each burst lasts from 30 to 90 seconds. Running wind sprints, lifting weights, and playing sports like soccer or tennis are examples of anaerobic exercise.

Here are some basic rules to follow in your exercise program:

- Train for the specific activity you are interested in. If you want to become a better swimmer, it makes no sense to ride a bicycle 100 miles a week. Instead, perform exercises that train the specific muscles involve in swimming.

- Vary your workouts. This is the central theme of a type of weight training called "periodized training," but it applies to fitness in general. Alternate aerobic activities with anaerobic activities from workout to workout, and alternate light-intensity days with heavy-intensity days. This will help you avoid muscle imbalances and prevent burnout.

- Push your body so that you get the benefit of each exercise. In weight training, this is called "overloading": you have to force your muscles to do more than they are used to doing, or else you won't get any real benefit from the exercise. Don't try to do too much too quickly. You don't want to wake up the day after you started exercising and not be able to get out of bed—you might end up saying, "Wait a minute, I'm too far out of shape. I'm not going to do this."

- Remember that your fitness will increase gradually. The gains will come eventually, but perhaps not in the first week or two. The key is to stick to a regular workout schedule. Conditioning comes down to common sense: You build gradually, but you need to keep your goal in mind, and the goal has to be realistic.

- Increase the frequency, intensity, and duration of your workouts so you don't hit a plateau and stop progressing. In most beginning weight programs, it is usually best to increase the weight used in any specific exercise by no more than five percent per week. For aerobic activities, you can progress by increasing the incline on a treadmill or stair-climber, for example, or by increasing the length of your session. Be sure to

spend a few workouts at each level before moving up to the next; this ensures that your body is ready to adapt.

Aerobic Conditioning

Subsequent chapters describe numerous specific stretching exercises in detail. Here, we will focus on aerobic fitness: what it is, how to achieve and maintain it, and how not to overdo it. Later sections in this chapter will introduce training with weights, the concept of cross-training, and how weight training and aerobic training can complement each other.

Many people equate aerobic training with an aerobics class, in which an instructor has a program of movements set to music that students follow. This is a fun and efficient way to get in shape, and there are many levels and types of aerobics classes to fit the needs of anyone who is interested.

There are many other ways to do aerobic conditioning, however. Perhaps you don't want to take a class with a bunch of strangers. Or you may like particular activities, like running, biking, or swimming, that you can do on your own. When you get right down to it, anything that gets your heart to pump harder for an extended period of time can improve aerobic fitness. Usually, this involves moving large muscle groups in a rhythmic fashion for at least 20 to 30 minutes.

You can use a machine: a stationary bike, a cross-country skiing machine, an elliptical trainer, or even an upper-body ergometer (where you pedal with your arms as if it were a bicycle). Walking or shoveling snow can also increase your heart rate for a sustained period. All of these activities make the heart stronger and able to pump more efficiently.

When your heart works at a higher level than normal, you achieve what is called "the aerobic effect," which is an improvement in your ability to oxygenate blood and move blood through the heart and lungs. This is a true measure of fitness and cardio-vascular health.

Your heart is not your brain, so it won't be able to distinguish what type of physical activity you are doing. It will, however, respond when it is being asked to work harder by moving blood faster, and, gradually, it will become more efficient at doing this. Exercises or exercise machines that work your upper and lower body simultaneously—cross-country skiing is a prime exam-ple—are the best for helping you reach your aerobic fitness goals because they make your heart work harder.

Still, you shouldn't do the same exercise over and over, even if it is aero-bically sound. It is best to vary your activities in order to avoid muscle imbalances or overuse injuries, as well as to keep you fresh. Ride your bike one day, lift weights another day, and play a sport another day. This is the concept of cross-training put into practice.

FREQUENCY

Experts recommend that you do some form of aerobic exercise at least three times a week, preferably on noncon-secutive days. A frequency of less than twice a week does not provide enough benefit, and a frequency of more than four times a week can overtax your body. The importance of rest cannot be overstated; as described in Chapter 7 on weight training, your body actually adapts and improves more on the days when you are not lifting weights than it does on the days you are in the gym. In addition, it is absolutely essential to give your muscles and joints a chance to recover between workouts. One school of thought suggests that five or even six workouts a week of moderate intensity will provide

increased benefit, but in the beginning at least, you should stick to three or four days a week.

Each session should last a minimum of 20 continuous minutes. If that is too much when you first start out, begin with 10 minutes of exercise and gradually build up to 12, 15, 18, and then 20 minutes. You should be com-fortable with 12 minutes of exercise before moving up to 15 minutes. Twenty minutes is considered the low threshold for achieving the aerobic effect; once you get to the point where you can keep going for that long, make it your minimum standard as well.

Studies have shown that once you pass 30 minutes of continuous activity, you gain little in the way of aerobic conditioning. You will, of course, burn more body fat and lose weight more quickly, the longer you are engaged in an activity.

INTENSITY

It is important to exercise at an intensity level vigorous enough to cause your heart rate to increase and your breathing to become more rapid. If you don't reach this intensity level, you won't reap the full benefits of the exercise.

Determining Your Target Heart Rate
According to the President's Council on Physical Fitness and Sports, perform the following calculations to find your target heart rate.

- Determine your maximum heart rate (MHR) by subtracting your age in years from 220.
- Multiply your MHR by 0.65 (65%) to determine your minimum aerobic training rate. Then multiply your MHR by 0.8 (80%) to determine your maximum aerobic training rate.

- The range of numbers between these minimum and maximum training rates, in heartbeats per minute, is your target heart rate.

For example, a 42-year-old person would subtract 42 from 220 to get 178, then multiply 178 by 0.65 to determine the lower threshold of the target zone, or 116. Then he/she would multiply 178 by 0.8 for the upper threshold, or 142. The target heart rate of a 42-year-old, then, is between 116 and 142 beats per minute.

As a general rule, beginners should aim for the lower threshold (65%) of their target heart rate, while more advanced people can work up to the 80% level. This is only a guide, however, and people with medical limitations should discuss this formula with their physician before starting any fitness program.

To determine whether your heart rate during exercise falls in your target heart rate range, perform the following steps:

- Count the number of pulse beats at your wrist or neck for 15 seconds, then multiply by four to find your current beats per minute. If you must interrupt your workout to check your heart rate, take your pulse within five seconds after interrupting, because your heartbeat starts to decrease once you stop moving.
- Compare your current beats per minute with your target zone. If your heartbeat is faster than the maximum, you may be overworking your heart and you may need to slow down your exercise.

Another way to gauge whether or not you may be pushing yourself too hard is to take the "talk test": your workout should make you sweat, but not make you so out of breath that you cannot talk.

Keep the following points in mind:

- Exercise that doesn't raise your heart rate to a certain level and keep it there for at least 20 minutes will not contribute significantly to your aerobic fitness.
- It will take some time to build your cardiovascular endurance. You need to start slowly and increase your activity gradually. It may take eight to 10 weeks before you see a dramatic improvement.
- Find an exercise routine that makes sense for you. Make sure that you enjoy it, that it fits into your schedule, and that it provides the benefits you want. If you find the routine awkward or difficult, you won't have the motivation to stick with it and you will be right back where you started.
- If you have any injuries or health problems, or if you are over 45 or pregnant, consult your physician before starting any exercise program. Exercise and diet can slow the aging process to a degree, but they cannot reverse it, and there is no dishonor in conceding that fact.

Precautions

There is such a thing as too much aerobic conditioning, and this can be problematic. Excessive aerobic training can have an oxidative effect, and too much oxidation harms the body. Oxidation is a process that degrades, like rusting metal; too much aerobic exercise breaks muscle down instead of building it up. Doctors believe that too much aerobic training can create metabolic problems and increase your risks of cancer and other diseases.

Exercise is like a medicine; too little yields only minimal benefits, and too much may cause serious damage. The wonderful thing about the human body is that it will tell you when you're doing too much—the message is in the form of injury or fatigue. If either of these occurs, take a break. Particularly with injuries, which are discussed in Chapter 4, "Err on the side of caution" is a phrase to live by. Fortunately, newer machines like elliptical trainers enable you to exercise even when you are recovering from an injury and cannot handle high-impact exercises. There is rarely a good excuse for not exercising.

WEIGHT TRAINING

How Muscles Work

To understand the benefits of weight training, it is helpful to understand how your muscles work and how they adapt to stress caused by resistance exercises.

When your muscles contract—which is what they do when you lift weights or exert force against some object— the muscle fibers contract and pull on tendons. This action moves the bones that rotate at the various joints in your body. You have three types of joints: uniaxial joints, which act like hinges (your elbows, for example); biaxial joints, which allow two types of movement in two directions (your wrists and ankles, for example); and multiaxial joints, which allow three types of movement (your shoulders, hips, and knees, for example).

Muscles are made up of thousands of cells called muscle fibers. The muscle fibers are stimulated to action by motor nerves that can control as few as one or as many as several hundred muscle fibers. The nerve-muscle combination is called a motor unit. The muscle fibers become excited when the nerves send a signal to the muscle in the form of an electric current that causes the release of acetylcholine, a chemical that causes the muscle fiber to contract. This action is called a twitch.

Muscle fibers are commonly classified as fast-twitch or slow-twitch. Fast-twitch muscle fibers develop force quickly and over a short period of time, while slow-twitch muscle fibers develop force more slowly and over a longer period of time. Not surprisingly, slow-twitch muscle fibers are what give you endurance and energy during, say, a distance race. Fast-twitch muscle fibers, on the other hand, are what allow you to sprint at full speed or perform other actions that are explosive but short in duration. Your muscles contain slow- and fast-twitch muscle fibers in varying proportions.

The Effect of Resistance Training

When you lift weights or perform other kinds of resistance training, you are increasing the size of your muscle fibers, a process known as hypertrophy. This helps you increase your strength. Interestingly, some studies have shown that fast-twitch muscle fibers show greater increases in size than slow-twitch fibers; this means that athletes with a higher percentage of fast-twitch fibers may have an advantage when it comes to resistance training. It also may explain why different athletes will increase muscle size in different proportions even if they are using the same training program.

Muscle-fiber increase from resistance training has been shown to be comparable in women and men, although it is often not as noticeable in women because they have a higher percentage of body fat than men, along with fewer hormones that help increase muscle size.

When you begin a weight training program like one of those described later in this book, your body generally requires about four to six weeks to make the overall adaptations to the new stresses it is undergoing. You may feel stronger within the first two weeks because your neurological system is making the adaptation more quickly, but your actual strength will take a little longer to increase. You also may not notice any significant difference in muscle size for the first month or two, even though you may feel yourself getting stronger.

As with aerobic exercise, you need to start slowly and build gradually when you are following a weight training program. You may not be lifting as much as the person next to you in the early stages, but you probably won't hit a plateau as early, either. And over the long term, your results will be the same or better.

CROSS-TRAINING

Assuming that overall fitness is your goal, cross-training is a logical way to achieve it. It is a simple concept: Include more than one type of exercise—ideally, several types—in your workout routine. This will have the dual effect of improving your fitness and protecting you from injury. Repeating the same exercises over time can cause overuse injuries, even to elite athletes. If you vary your activities, you will give more and different muscles a workout and avoid muscle imbalances.

The term *cross-training* became popular within the last two decades, but the concept has actually been around far longer among elite athletes and others with a desire to break up their exercise routine.

A good cross-training program includes aerobic conditioning, flexibility, strength training, and perhaps some type of sports activity. This could entail biking, running, swimming, stair-climbing, or other aerobic activity, combined with stretching or yoga and weight lifting or other types of resistance training. The idea is to work different muscles in different ways to achieve overall fitness. Running or bicycling can get your lower body in great shape and improve your cardiovascular fitness, but it won't exercise the muscles in your upper body. Swimming and cross-country skiing, on the other hand, provide a more general workout and have the additional benefit of being low-impact exercises.

Cardiovascular exercises like the ones described above should be the basic building blocks of your cross-training program, but they should not be the only exercises you do. Flexibility and strength exercises are as important for your overall fitness, because they prepare your muscles for the stresses of different types of athletic maneuvers. For example, if you ride a bicycle, then run a few miles, you will find it very taxing on your muscles. This is because you use your leg muscles differently for biking than for running, and your body adapts differently to each form of exercise. If you combine activities on a regular basis, you will find that your body adapts much better to other stresses that you place on it.

Aerobic Training vs. Weight Training

As described earlier in this chapter, aerobic training and weight training are both vital parts of any exercise program. But aerobic exercise is steady, consistent motion, while weight training requires short, explosive movements. How do the two affect each other?

Studies have shown that weight training will not appreciably improve your muscles' aerobic capacity—but it won't decrease it, either. In fact, weight training may actually improve short-term muscle endurance for athletes such as cyclists or distance runners.

Aerobic or endurance training, on the other hand, will increase your aerobic capacity, but it won't increase strength—and in many cases, it may actually decrease strength. For example, a sprinter wouldn't train by jogging a few miles per day instead of running sprints, because jogging could decrease the development of fast-twitch muscle fibers that are required for running at high speeds.

Some kinds of weight training can have aerobic benefits. One is "super circuit training," in which you perform one set of a weight exercise, then immediately jump rope, do jumping jacks, or ride a stationary bike before the next weight set. Similarly, there are complex exercises that involve two distinct parts; for example, you would do 10 repetitions with a barbell in a squat position and immediately follow that with several lunges or jumps. These types of exercises should only be done under proper supervision and with full instruction beforehand.

4

Safety and Avoiding Injury

Injuries can and do happen to people who are physically active. Sometimes they are the result of an unavoidable accident, but the most common ones are "overuse" injuries, which are usually the result of trying to do too much too soon or overreaching your abilities.

When you first begin a new activity or program, aches and pains are normal. They are also normal when the intensity of an activity or program is increased. Proper stretching before and after the activity, however, can help prevent much of the soreness. Nevertheless, actual pain—rather than soreness—may indicate an injury, and you should see a doctor about it.

The most common types of athletic injuries are muscle pulls, strains, and sprains. These affect your tendons, muscles, and ligaments and can occur when you don't stretch properly before working out. Of course, they can happen even if you do stretch, especially if you are involved in sports that require you to pivot or make sudden, rapid movements or if you are pushing yourself too hard in the weight room. Nevertheless, it pays to prepare your muscles and joints before you place stress on them, and to help them recover when you are finished working out.

WARM-UP AND COOLDOWN

For the sake of your heart, your muscles, and your motivation, you need to fashion a workout routine that includes three distinct phases: warm-up, exercise, and cooldown.

The Warm-Up

A survey of members of the orthopedist group Professional Team Physicians revealed that overuse and over-extension injuries are two of the leading injury categories they see in athletes. Warming up properly can help protect against these types of injuries.

A good warm-up takes only five to 10 minutes, but the benefits are significant. It allows you to ease your body into an activity by sending more blood to your muscles. Think of it as a wake-up call to your muscles: You're telling them what they can expect in the next hour or so.

A good warm-up raises the temperature of your muscles and tissues, increases your metabolic rate (the number of calories your body burns to maintain normal body functions), prepares your cardiovascular system for work by speeding up your heart rate, and decreases muscle tension.

There are many ways to warm up. You can walk around or perform some other low-intensity aerobic work like light jogging on a treadmill, jumping rope, or riding an exercise bike—any activity that makes you start to sweat and gets your heart pumping and your blood circulating faster.

Once you feel your body is warmer and your muscles loosen up a bit, do some stretching exercises; examples of these can be found in Chapter 6. You should take the time to stretch important areas of your body—calves, hamstrings, quadriceps, back, and shoulders—without rushing. Stretching after your muscles are warmed up is also more effective than stretching when your muscles are cold.

If possible, a warm-up should be geared to the specific activity you are planning. For instance, if you are going to ride a stationary bike, you could warm up by riding easily for a few minutes, then focusing on stretching your quadriceps and hamstrings.

The Cooldown

Cooling down is no less important in your training routine than warming up. Whatever activity you are engaged in, you need to allow adequate time for your body to make the transition from being stressed to being at rest.

Once you have finished your workout, the worst thing that you can do is to stop moving entirely, for instance by heading straight back to work and sitting at your desk. This will cause the buildup of lactic acid in your muscles, which can cause soreness. Spend five minutes tapering off your activity at the end of your workout. For instance, if you are on the treadmill, slow the machine down before you are ready to finish; if you are running, biking, or swimming, slow the activity down near the end. You can even walk around for a few minutes. The point is to keep moving and keep your blood flowing.

The other part of cooling down is stretching. This helps your muscles recover from the stresses you have placed on them. Stretch thoroughly, paying particular attention to the muscles you used most during your workout.

Rehydrate yourself by drinking water, even if you do not feel thirsty, because your body has lost fluids that need to be replaced. If you have a previously injured area or one that feels sore, apply ice to it for 10 to 15 minutes in order to reduce inflammation.

Breathing

Breathing is something you do without thinking. When you are exercising, however, you may have to think about it a little, at least at first. All forms of exercise demand that you use proper breathing technique, which can help increase blood flow and remove lactic acid from your muscles. Correct breathing is also important when you are stretching, because it increases blood flow to the muscles, thereby improving their elasticity.

In general, your breathing should be slow, rhythmic, and relaxed. Inhale through your nose and exhale through your mouth. Expand your abdomen when you inhale. When you are lifting a weight, exhale as you push the weight upward or forward. During aerobic exercise, you may find that your breathing becomes more rapid and difficult, particularly if you are just starting out; concentrate on breathing as slowly and naturally as possible.

CONQUERING THE ELEMENTS

Hot and cold weather should not be used as excuses to avoid working out, but you shouldn't try to conquer these elements without knowing the risks involved. Both conditions require you to arm yourself with the proper clothing and gear, and to modify your workouts as well.

Cold Weather

The "What To Wear" section in Chapter 1 contains the suggestion to wear layers to keep warm when exercising in cold weather. In addition, you should check conditions to make sure they are safe— this applies especially to runners, joggers, and bicyclists, who may encounter ice or snow on the roads. During the winter, it gets dark earlier, so be sure to wear reflective material on your clothing when exercising late in the day.

Exercising in cold weather can aggravate the symptoms of asthma. Wearing a scarf over your mouth and nose can help, as can breathing in through your nose instead of your mouth, since your nose warms the air before it reaches your lungs.

Stretching is even more important in cold weather, since your muscles tend to be tighter. This means that stretching after your workout is also crucial, even if you finish your workout and immediately go indoors.

Hot Weather

When exercising on a hot, humid day, the most important thing to do is to drink plenty of fluids. Because your thirst mechanism does not always tell you when and how much you need to drink, you may already be dehydrated by the time you feel thirsty, and heat exhaustion may result.

In general, you should drink a quart of fluid for every pound of body fluid you lose during exercise—enough so that your urine is light-colored and not dark yellow. You should drink water at least every 15 minutes while exercising on hot, humid days. Avoid caffeinated drinks and alcohol before (and, certainly, during!) exercise, since these liquids can cause you to lose extra fluids.

During the summer, plan your outdoor exercise early in the morning or late in the afternoon to avoid exposure during the hottest hours of the day. A little sun is good for everybody, but too much can cause problems.

Wear loose-fitting clothing made from material that breathes (like cotton), and wear a hat or sun visor to keep direct sunlight off your head and face.

If you are working out or playing sports on artificial turf or another man-made surface, you are more susceptible to heat illness and should take extra care to stay cool. Pour cold water over your head or soak your hat in cold water before putting it on.

Signs of Heat Illness and How to Avoid It

There are three levels of heat illness: cramps, heat exhaustion, and heat stroke. As the words imply, these conditions progress from mild discomfort to a potentially life-threatening illness.

Cramps occur when there is not enough blood flow to the leg muscles and the muscles' balance of water and electrolytes, such as sodium, potassium, and calcium, is upset. This usually affects the lower legs and abdominal muscles. Treatment of heat-related muscle cramps includes stopping strenuous activity and moving to a cooler place; stretching and then massaging afflicted muscle groups, followed by applying ice; and replenishment of fluids with water, a sports drink, or fruit juice.

Heat exhaustion is caused by dehydration. Symptoms include chills, light-headedness, dizziness, heavy perspiration, cool and pale or flushed skin, headache, and nausea. If you experience any of these symptoms, stop your activity immediately. Move to a cool place and remove excess clothing. Rehydrate with fluids and sprinkle your body with cool water. Seek medical assistance immediately.

Heat stroke is a medical emergency caused by a failure of the body's thermoregulatory system. It may be fatal if not treated. Its symptoms are similar to heat exhaustion, but may also include disorientation, loss of consciousness, and, ultimately, seizures. You may also stop sweating and experience an irregular or rapid heartbeat. Severe dehydration can damage the brain and other organs of the body.

For heat stroke, seek medical assistance as soon as possible. Immediate treatment includes either cool baths or ice packs placed near large arteries, such as at those in the neck and armpits. Fluids should be taken immediately.

Here are some tips for avoiding heat illness:

- Drink fluids 30 minutes before exercise and every 15 minutes during exercise. After exercise, drink more fluids.
- Don't exercise in hot weather if you are not already in good physical shape. Build up your tolerance to hot weather by starting with short workouts.
- If you have a medical condition that may affect your tolerance to heat, such as diabetes or high blood

pressure, consult your physician before exercising outdoors in hot weather.

- If possible, move your activities indoors. If this is not possible, work out in the early morning or late afternoon/early evening, when it is cooler.
- Be sure to stretch and warm up— even though it is warm outside, the heat will not automatically make your muscles loose and limber without stretching.
- If you experience any of the symptoms of heat exhaustion or heat stroke listed above, particularly dizziness or light-headedness, stop immediately, rest, and rehydrate.

Protection Against the Sun

More attention has been paid to skin cancer in recent years, and rightly so. Repeated sunburns and exposure to direct sunlight can cause irreparable damage to the skin of anyone who spends a lot of time playing or training outdoors.

Two types of ultraviolet light, UVA and UVB, can be harmful to the skin. UVA light damages the deeper skin layer and may lead to melanoma (malignant skin tumor). Sunburn is usually the result of overexposure to UVB rays. UVB light damages the superficial layer of the skin and can cause carcinoma, the most common form of skin cancer. UVB light also causes cataracts, which cloud the lens of the eye, causing impaired vision.

The SPF (sun protection factor) number on sunscreen products gives a theoretical measure of UVB protection. It indicates the amount of time it takes skin to burn. If burning would occur in 20 minutes with no protection, wearing a sunscreen with an SPF of 10 would delay burning until 200 minutes have elapsed. Since sweat and other moisture can reduce the effectiveness of sunscreen, many dermatologists recommend waterproof sunscreens.

Some sunscreens offer protection against both UVA and UVB rays. Sunscreens containing PARSOL 1789 may give better protection against UVA rays.

Even if you use sunscreen with a high SPF number, keep in mind that sunscreen may rub or wear off during activity, requiring reapplication.

Here are some tips to prevent sunburn and other sun-related problems:

- Use a sunscreen with an SPF rating of at least 15.
- Apply sunscreen liberally. Make sure all exposed areas are covered, including the tops of your feet if they are going to be exposed.
- Even on overcast days, the sun's rays can still have adverse effects.
- If you are working out at high altitudes, take into account that you are getting increased exposure to the sun.
- Wear sunglasses to protect your eyes from UVB light, which is a cause of cataracts.

OVERTRAINING

People who push themselves hard at work tend to do the same when they work out. Your body, however, may be much more fragile than you think it is. If you ask it to work too hard over a period of time, it will rebel. Pushing yourself may get you to a higher level of fitness, but your body may begin to shut down if you push it too hard, and this can nullify many of the gains you have made. There may be adverse psychological effects as well. In other words, "no pain, no gain" is not always the best philosophy.

Overtraining is the name given to this phenomenon, and there are recog-

nizable symptoms. These include altered eating habits, difficulty sleeping, nausea, mood swings, sore and tired muscles, depression, lack of motivation, and frequent illnesses. You get the feeling you are not benefiting as much from your workout as you normally do.

If you experience any of these symptoms, you should take stock of your training routine. Talk to a trainer or physical fitness professional, or consult your physician. Examine your workout schedule and try to schedule extra rest between workouts. You won't get out of shape by taking a few days off; instead, you will feel fresh and rejuvenated and ready to return to your workouts with a new attitude.

How to Avoid Overtraining

- Listen to your body. You should feel better after a workout, not worse. If you don't feel better, and this happens consistently, you should consider making some changes in your routine.
- Rest! When you are exercising, muscle tissue breaks down. If you push your muscles constantly, you run the risk of wearing the muscle tissue down.
- Stay hydrated. Dehydration can cause extra fatigue and overheat your body.
- Maintain a healthy diet and get enough sleep. Nothing can sabotage your exercise routine more than not eating enough food, or eating the wrong foods, and not getting enough sleep. Eat complex carbohydrates, such as pasta and cereal, along with fruits, vegetables, and adequate protein.
- Take painkillers when needed, but remember that they are masking pain, not treating it. If there is a problem underlying the pain, get it checked out before it turns into a bigger problem.

- Plan a workout or workouts that you like. If boredom is creeping into your routine, make changes. This will help you stay fresh and motivated.
- Vary your routine by including different activities. This is the concept behind cross-training, and it is a good way to avoid overtraining.

DEALING WITH INJURIES

Injuries are a part of sports and a part of exercising. Even if you start your workout program gradually and slowly increase its intensity, you may find that you are fatigued by the end of your workout and are sore the next day. This is normal; it is your body's way of adapting to the new stresses being placed on it. The question is, when is it soreness and when is it a sign of injury?

This is not the time to be a hero—untreated injuries only become worse!

For general soreness—which you are guaranteed to experience the day after your first workout—it is often wise to pull back a little and lower your intensity. For example, if you did one set of several exercises during your first workout and had minimal soreness/stiffness, you would probably do one set again in your second workout. If you did one set the first day and felt no soreness at all, you might do two sets the second day. If you felt very sore after the first day, however, you might wait until the soreness went away before resuming, and even then you should probably lower the amount of weight.

RICE

Fortunately, many of the most common injuries can be treated at home, after you've assessed the severity of the injury and have determined that medical advice is not required. For strains and sprains, the guidelines most often recommended are easily remembered by the acronym **RICE**, which stands for Rest, Ice, Compression, Elevation.

For bruises, strains, and sprains, RICE is usually what a doctor recommends. Although it is sometimes necessary to immobilize an injury with an elastic wrap, brace, sling, splint, or crutches, RICE is the most common and effective follow-up, a therapy that every athlete should know how to use. Fortunately, it is easy to remember and simple to apply:

Rest, which means refraining from strenuous activities and staying off your feet as much as possible. Just putting your body weight on a sprained ankle or strained calf muscle can slow your rehabilitation.

Ice, which causes arteries and veins to constrict and reduces pain and swelling. Apply ice for about 15 minutes as soon after an injury as possible. Repeat applications for two or three more days, 10 to 15 minutes at a time and three times a day.

Compression, or wrapping, which holds the injured area or joint in place. This can reduce swelling and irritation.

Elevation, which also helps reduce swelling. Raise the affected area to a level higher than your heart and keep it there while you are resting. This will decrease blood flow to the area.

RICE is simple to remember and effective for treating minor injuries, providing you practice it diligently. It can speed your return to the gym or road.

Taping and Wrapping

Taping and wrapping an injured muscle or joint can allow you to continue working out while you are rehabilitating a minor injury. It should never, however, take the place of advice from your physician or orthopedist.

Taping and wrapping provide support and compression for an injured area. Wraps and braces made of elastic or neoprene can be applied with a few simple rules.

Above all, do not make the wrap too tight. It should provide support but not cut off the blood supply. This takes some practice if you are taping or applying an elastic bandage. Numbness, tingling, and swelling are signs that you may have taped or wrapped too tightly. Wrapping too loosely, on the other hand, can defeat the purpose of wrapping.

Use braces or wraps that do not have seams or straps that can chafe or irritate the skin.

In psychological terms, the wrap should remind you that one of your joints or muscles is not 100% fit and that you do, in fact, have an injury. This alone is useful.

Taping and wrapping will not heal an injury. But with time and the proper treatments (like RICE), it can help you get back to exercising sooner. The most important step to take if you are injured (or think you are) is to seek medical advice from your physician, physical therapist, or certified trainer before you embark on any treatment course.

When to See a Doctor and What to Ask

When deciding whether to seek medical attention for an injury, you should err on the side of caution. The President's Council on Physical Fitness and Sports recommends seeing a doctor under the following circumstances:

- The pain is extreme or persistent.
- You've suffered trauma to a joint, possibly affecting the underlying connective tissue.
- An injury does not heal in a reasonable period of time.
- You develop an infection or fever.
- You're unsure about the severity of the injury.

It's easy to forget to ask all of the questions you want to ask when you see a physician, and it can be frustrating when you think of the questions you would have liked to ask after you've left the doctor's office. The Association of Professional Team Physicians recommends asking the following questions:

- What is the diagnosis?
- What activities should I avoid, and for how long?
- What activities or exercises are helpful?
- Will it help to apply ice or heat?
- Should I wear a brace or protective bandage?
- Should I take medication for pain or inflammation?
- When can I return to my usual activities?
- Is there a way to avoid similar injuries in the future?
- If I am not getting better in a few weeks, should I return or have further diagnostic tests?
- Are there any complications I should look out for?

5

Exercise and Pregnancy

Studies have found that pregnant women who exercise regularly can reap benefits like decreased stress and depression, better posture, better digestion, and less constipation. They have also found that women who exercise typically have faster postpartum recoveries.

Pregnant women should be sure to consult their obstetrician before embarking on an exercise routine, even if they have exercised regularly before becoming pregnant. Once exercise has been approved by your doctor, you should begin cautiously and avoid any activities that cause pain, shortness of breath, or excessive fatigue.

If you are exercising while pregnant, you may need to increase your daily caloric intake above what is normal for pregnant women. You should also make sure to increase your fluid intake to avoid dehydration and overheating.

The American College of Obstetricians and Gynecologists recommends that healthy pregnant women do low-impact, cardiovascular activities for 30 minutes at least three times a week.

Here are some tips to develop a safe and effective fitness routine while pregnant:

- Be sure to warm up and stretch before you exercise, and be sure to cool down when you are done. Cooling down allows blood to return to your heart and uterus.
- Whatever activity you choose, use fluid, controlled movements rather than fast, jerky movements.
- Avoid high-impact exercises like running and aerobics. These can stress your joints and lead to fatigue, nausea, and discomfort. Instead, do low-impact activities like walking, swimming, and stationary cycling.
- Weight training can help maintain posture and muscle tone, particularly in the shoulders, upper back, and abdomen. Strengthening upper back muscles can help after birth when you are picking up or breast-feeding your baby. To avoid undue stress on your muscles, use light weights and more repetitions instead of heavy weights and few repetitions.

6

Stretching

Stretching should be a fundamental part of your workout routine, but it is often the one element that is either forgotten or intentionally skipped. You may occasionally hear someone claim that he/she never stretches and has never pulled a muscle, but this is a rare exception (or an outright exaggeration).

Stretching helps you in two ways: (1) It improves flexibility, which gets your muscles and joints loose and ready for exercise, and (2) it helps prevent injury. It should be done before and after a workout, but you can also stretch when you aren't working out, just to keep yourself flexible.

For people with certain types of injuries, stretching exercises are often prescribed to be performed every day, whether or not a workout is scheduled. If you have suffered an injury, consult your orthopedist or physical therapist about which stretches are helpful in your rehabilitation (and which could be harmful).

WHY SHOULD YOU STRETCH?

Here are some of the benefits of stretching as a regular part of your workout routine:

- It increases your range of motion, improving coordination and making it easier to perform your workout exercises.
- It reduces muscle tension and soreness.
- It decreases the risk of injury. When you stretch your muscles, they actually lengthen and are thus better prepared to withstand stress and strain.
- It improves your balance and agility.
- It aids in the circulation of blood to your muscles.
- It heightens your sense of your own body and how your muscles and joints work together, a phenomenon known as "proprioception."
- It may make menstruation less painful for women.

SOME RULES FOR STRETCHING

Most of us believe that being active means putting our bodies in motion—and quickly. We don't like to be bothered to relax, move slowly, and breathe properly. But to get the most out of stretching (and out of your workout), you need to do these things.

When you begin stretching, keep the following points in mind:

- Do a brief warm-up before you stretch. This may seem to fly in the face of logic, but it is important! You need to get the blood flowing to your muscles before you stretch them, or you run the risk of tearing them. The 5-to-10–minute warm-up can be any exercise that raises your heart rate and gets you sweating, like walking, jogging, or riding a stationary bike.
- Go slowly and ease into each stretch. If you feel any pain in a muscle, pull back.
- Hold each stretch for at least 15 seconds—longer, if possible. You will find that you can hold stretches longer the more you do them.
- Use a smooth, fluid motion. Never bounce when you stretch, and don't use a jerky motion. This will increase the risk of tearing muscles or tendons.
- Breathe! Just as you do when you are lifting a weight, you need to breathe slowly and regularly while stretching in order to stay loose and relaxed.
- Stretch all the major muscle groups, even if you will be focusing on a particular group of muscles in your workout. Move from one area of your body to another. For example, you could begin with your shoulders, neck, and upper back and move downward to your arms and hip flexors, then to your quadriceps and

hamstrings, and finally to your shins and calves. Figure out a sequence and make it your routine.
- Don't shortchange yourself on stretching. Take your time and be thorough; it usually won't take more than 10 minutes anyway. You might want to use those 10 minutes to visualize what you're about to do in your workout or sport.
- Stretch before and after your workout. Afterward, stretching as part of your cooldown will help rid your muscles of lactic acid that can cause cramping.
- If you have a joint injury or muscle pull, don't stretch the injured area. Consult a physician, who will probably refer you to a physical therapist who can recommend specific stretches to help you rehabilitate your injury.

STRETCHES FOR DIFFERENT AREAS OF THE BODY

Obviously, you won't have the time or—let's face it—the inclination to perform all these stretches. Pick out the ones that seem right for you and try them, then incorporate them into your workout routine. Remember: Stretching should not be a chore, so make efficient use of your stretching time by doing only the stretches you need, clearing your head, and focusing on the workout you are about to do.

Head and Neck Stretches
Chin Circles
Tuck your chin back toward your throat. With your chin, draw a circle outward and around, starting and ending with your chin tucked back toward your throat. Repeat five times. Reverse the direction of the circle. Repeat five times.

Head Lift

Lie on your back on the floor, bend your knees, lift your head, and lace the fingers of both hands behind your head. Use your arms to pull your head forward slowly. You should feel the stretch in the back of your neck. Hold the stretch for a count of five. Slowly return to the starting position. Repeat five times.

Head Rotation to the Side

Slowly turn your head to one side. Hold the stretch for a count of three. Slowly return to the starting position. Then turn your head to the other side. Hold the stretch for a count of three. Return to the starting position. Repeat five to 10 times. Try doing a set of this exercise two or three times a day.

Horizontal Neck Tilt

Slowly tilt your head to the side. Stop when you feel a strain, and be careful not to go so far that your ear touches your shoulder. Hold the stretch for a count of three. Slowly tilt your head back to the starting position. Then tilt your head to the other side. Hold the stretch for a count of three. Return to the starting position. Repeat five to 10 times. Try doing a set of this exercise two or three times a day.

Vertical Neck Tilt

Slowly tilt your head back until you are looking up at the ceiling. Hold the stretch for a count of three. Then slowly tilt your head back to the starting position. Lower your head until you are looking down at the floor. Hold the stretch for a count of three. Return to the starting position. Repeat five to 10 times. Try doing a set of this exercise two or three times a day.

Back and Chest Stretches

Back and Arm Stretches

1. Standing, link your hands together behind the middle of your back. Rotate your elbows inward while you straighten your arms. Repeat four or five times.
2. Standing, link your hands together behind your back. Lift your arms up until you feel a nice stretch. Hold for 10 to 20 seconds. Repeat as often as you like.
3. Standing, reach your arms behind you at shoulder level, and grab something—both sides of a doorway, for example. Lean forward and straighten your arms. Hold for 10 seconds. Slowly return to the starting position. Repeat as often as you like.

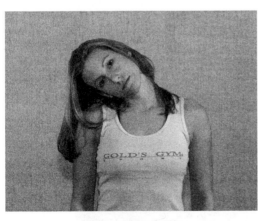

Horizontal Neck Tilt

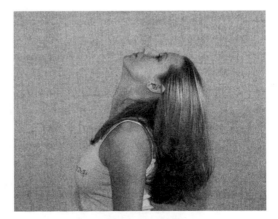

Vertical Neck Tilt

Back Stretches

1. Get onto your hands and knees on the floor. Sink down until you are resting your buttocks on your heels, with your knees together. Lean your head forward, with your forehead moving toward the floor and your hands next to your face. Hold this stretch for as long as you like.

2. Get onto your hands and knees on the floor. Sink down until you are resting your buttocks on your heels, with your knees together. Reach your arms forward and relax. To feel the stretch on one side or the other, you can move your hips. Hold this stretch for a minute or so. Return to the starting position. Repeat a few times.

Bending Side to Side

Stand with your arms at your sides. Bend from the waist toward one side and then the other. Repeat up to 50 times.

The Cat

Get onto your hands and knees on the floor. Start with your back flat, and keep your arms straight. Let your lower back sink as far as possible, without raising your head, to a concave position. Then slowly arch your back until you're curled in a convex position. Return to the starting position. Repeat 15 to 20 times.

Lower Back Stretch

Lie on your back on the floor and relax your back muscles. Slowly bring your

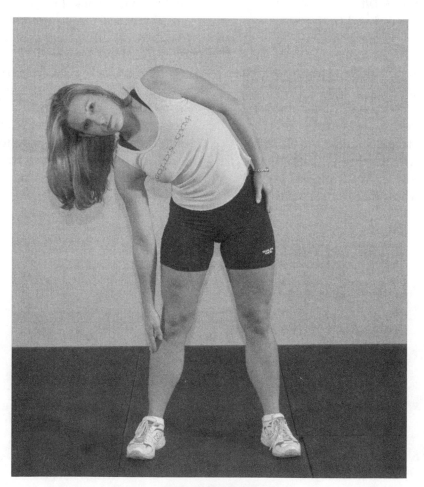

Bending Side to Side

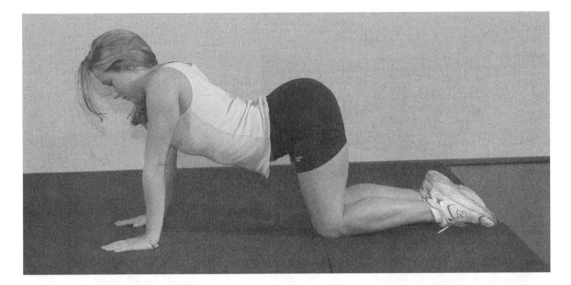

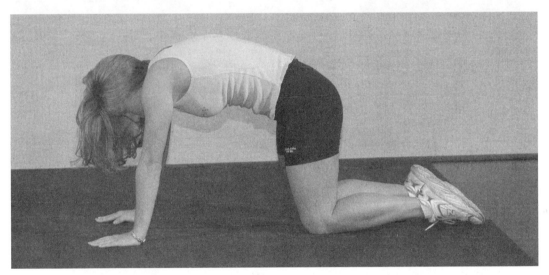

The Cat

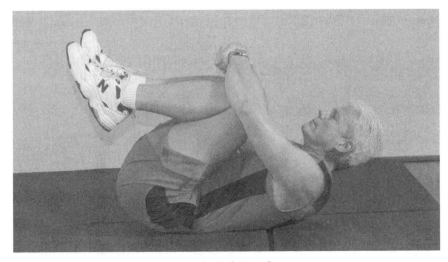

Lower Back Stretch

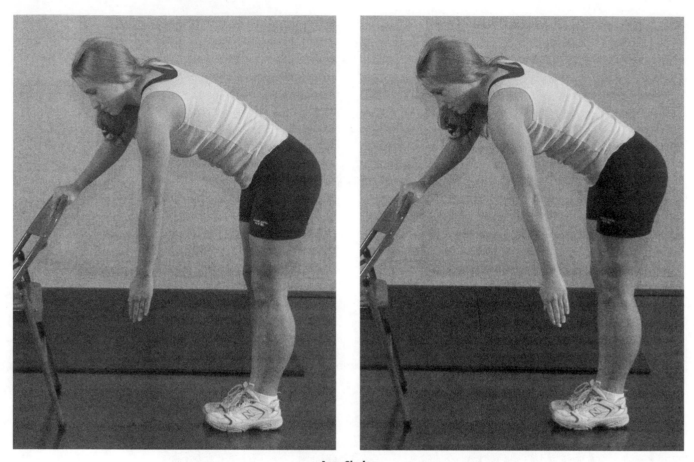

Arm Circles

knees up to your chest. Curl your arms around your knees. Hold for 15 to 20 seconds. Return to the starting position. Repeat 10 times. You can also do this exercise raising only one leg at a time.

Stretches for Arms, Shoulders, and Wrists

Arm Circles
Stand behind a chair and grasp the back of the chair with one hand. Bend forward at the waist. To protect your back, you should bend your knees slightly. The free arm should hang down, and your shoulder blade should be lowered. Swing your free arm in small circles. Repeat the motion and change the direction of the circles. Repeat the exercise with your other arm.

Arm Stretch
Extend your left arm in front of you. With your right hand, grasp your left elbow. Look over your left shoulder, and pull your left elbow toward your right shoulder. Hold for 15 seconds. Slowly return to the starting position. Repeat two or three times. Repeat the exercise with your right arm.

Flexing Wrist
With your arms extended in front of you, flex your wrists and stretch your fingers up toward the ceiling, then down toward the floor. Repeat 10 to 20 times.

Pendulum Swing (illustrated on p. 38)
Lie on your stomach along the edge of a bench, with one arm hanging over

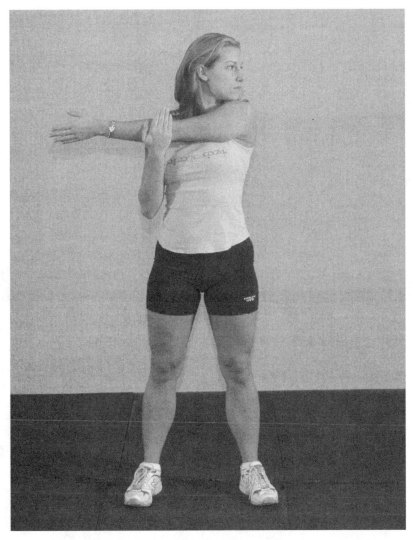

Arm Stretch

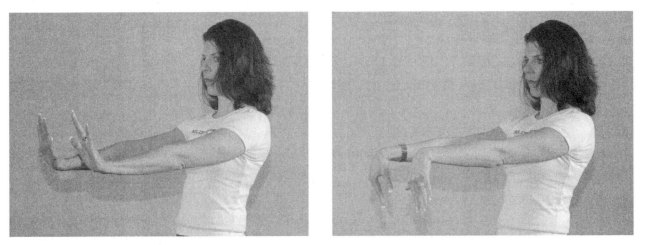

Flexing Wrist

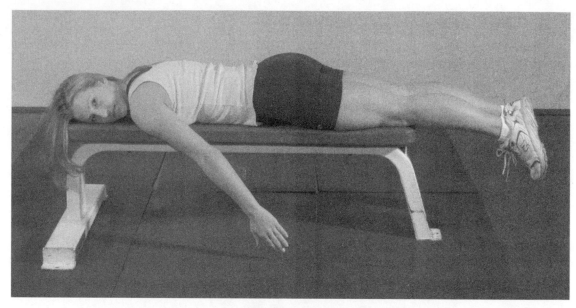

Pendulum Swing

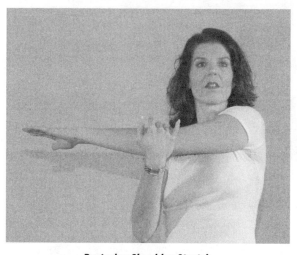

Posterior Shoulder Stretch

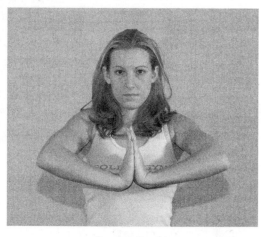

Praying Hands

the side. Relax your shoulder, arm, and hand, and make sure your shoulder blade is lowered. Slowly swing your arm to the front and to the back. If you experience any pain, restrict the sweep of the swing. Repeat the exercise with your other arm.

Posterior Shoulder Stretch

Standing, extend your left arm in front of you at shoulder height. Grasp your left elbow with your right hand and pull the arm across your body. You should feel the tension in the back of your shoulder. Slowly return to the starting position. Repeat two or three times, then repeat with your right arm.

Praying Hands

Stand straight, with your hands together in a praying position close to your chest. Raise your elbows until you feel the stretch in your forearms. Hold for 10 to 15 seconds. Slowly return to the starting position. Next, place the backs of your hands together, with your fingers pointing down. Hold for 10 to 15 seconds.

Raised Arm Stretches

1. Standing erect, raise your arms straight above your head. Rise up on your toes and clench your fists. Hold for 10 to 15 seconds. Maintaining this position, spread your fingers

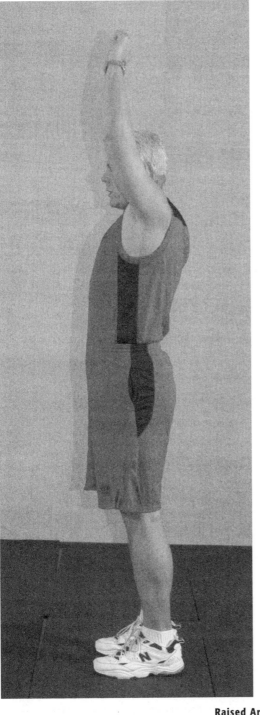 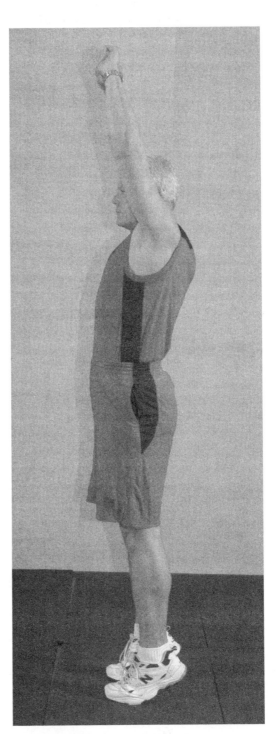

Raised Arm Stretch 1

apart. Rotate your hands in one direction five times, then in the other direction five times.

2. Standing erect, raise your arms above your head. Lace your fingers together, palms turned upward. Push your arms back and up, until you feel the stretch in your arms, shoulders, and back. Hold for 10 to 15 seconds. Slowly lower your arms to the starting position. Repeat four to six times.

Rotating Wrist

With your arm extended in front of you, make a fist and rotate your hand from the wrist. Do this in one direction 10 times, then in the other direction 10 times, about one-quarter turn each. Next, open your fist, and rotate your hand with the fingers extended.

Shoulder Blade Crunch

Lace your fingers together behind your head. Move your elbows back to pinch your shoulder blades together. Hold for three seconds, then return your elbows to the starting position. Repeat three times.

Shoulder Blade Stretch

Standing or sitting, reach across your chest and try to grasp your shoulder blades with your opposite hands.

Drop your chin toward your chest. Inhale and hold onto your shoulder blades for 15 seconds. You should feel the stretch along the border of your shoulder blades. Repeat five to 10 times.

Shoulder and Upper Arm Stretch

Standing, grasp the back of your left shoulder with your right hand. Hold your right elbow in your left hand, and gently pull the elbow to the left, until you feel a nice stretch. Repeat the exercise with your left arm. Perform three times with each arm.

Extended Arm Stretches

1. Extend one arm straight in front of you, with the wrist flexed and the

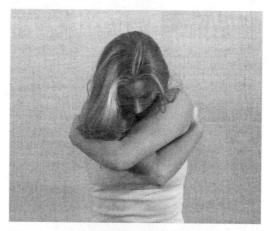

Shoulder Blade Stretch

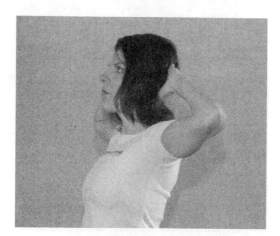

Shoulder Blade Crunch

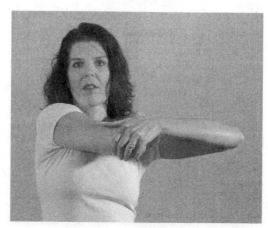

Shoulder and Upper Arm Stretch

fingers pointing up. Grasp the hand and thumb with the other hand, and pull the wrist back. Hold for 10 to 15 seconds. Relax. Repeat 10 to 20 times. Next, flex the wrist and point the fingers down. Grasp the back of the hand and thumb with the other hand, and pull the wrist inward. Hold for 10 to 15 seconds. Relax. Repeat 10 to 20 times. Repeat the exercise with your other arm.

2. Standing, extend one arm straight in front of you. Flex the wrist and point the fingers down until you feel a stretch across the top of the forearm. Next, flex the wrist and point the fingers up, until you feel a stretch across the bottom of the forearm. Repeat the exercise with your other arm. Perform five times with each arm.

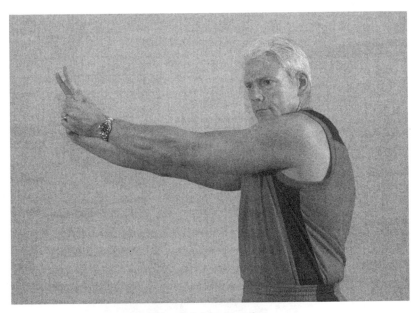

Extended Arm Stretch 1

Stretching Fingers
Extend your arms in front of you. Spread the fingers of each hand, trying to reach maximum extension. Hold for five seconds. Curl your fingers in, without clenching. Keep your fingers curled for five seconds. Repeat four to six times.

Triceps and Shoulder Stretch
Standing, raise your arms straight above your head. Grasp the elbow of one arm with the hand of the other. Pull that elbow behind your head until you feel a nice stretch. Hold for 10 to 15 seconds. Slowly return to the starting position. Repeat two or three times. Repeat the exercise with your other arm.

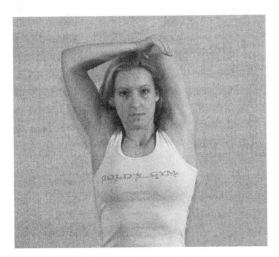

Triceps and Shoulder Stretch

of forearm muscles. Repeat the exercise with your other arm. Perform three times with each arm.

Wrist Extensor Stretch
Standing or sitting, extend your arm in front of you slightly lower than shoulder height, keeping your elbow straight and palm down. Using your opposite hand, bend the hand down so that your fingers are pointing toward the floor. You should feel the stretch in your wrist and the outside group

Wrist Flexor and Elbow Extensor Stretch
Standing or sitting, raise your arm in front of you slightly lower than shoulder height, keeping your elbow straight and palm up. Using the opposite hand, bend the hand down so that your fingers are pointing toward the floor. You should feel the stretch in

the tendons of the wrist and the inside group of forearm muscles. Repeat the exercise with your other arm. Perform three times with each arm.

Leg Stretches

Hamstring Stretches

1. Lie on your back on the floor, with your right leg straight in front of you and your left leg bent. Grasp your left ankle and slowly raise and straighten your leg. Keep your lower back on the floor. Hold for 10 seconds. Relax. Repeat five to 10 times. Repeat the exercise with your right leg.

2. Lie on your back on the floor. Lean forward to grasp the outside of your left ankle. Pull the leg toward your chest. Hold for 15 to 30 seconds. Slowly return to the starting position. Repeat four to five times. Repeat the exercise with your right leg.

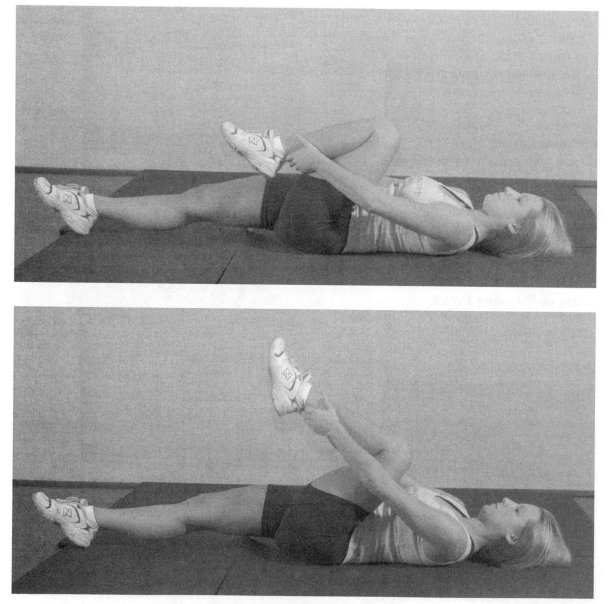

Hamstring Stretch 1

3. Sit on an exercise table or bench, with one leg bent at the knee and resting over the edge and the other leg extended straight in front of you. Keeping your back straight, reach forward with outstretched arms. Hold for 15 to 30 seconds. Return your arms to the starting position. Repeat six to 10 times. Repeat the exercise with your other leg.

Leg Swoops (illustrated on p. 44)

Get onto your hands and knees on the floor. Bend your head down, and bend your left knee forward until you touch your forehead. Next, as you raise your head, stretch the leg straight out behind you. Return to the starting position. Repeat 10 times. Repeat the exercise with your right leg.

Quadriceps and Hamstring Stretch

(illustrated on p. 45)

Loop a belt around your right foot and lie on your stomach. Using your right hand, pull the belt over your shoulder and bend the knee, being careful not to arch your back. Hold for 30 to 60 seconds. Relax. Repeat four

to five times. Repeat the exercise with your left leg.

Quadriceps Stretches (illustrated on p. 45)

1. Lie on your left side on the floor, resting the side of your head in your left hand. Stretch your left leg out on the floor. Grasp your right foot behind you, and pull the heel toward your buttocks. Hold for 10 to 20 seconds. Relax. Repeat four to five times. Repeat the exercise while lying on your right side and grasping your left foot.

2. Sit on the floor with one leg bent, touching the heel of the foot to the opposite hip. You can bend the other leg as well, or leave it straight in front of you. Hold for 10 to 20 seconds. Repeat four to five times. Repeat the exercise with your other leg.

3. Sit on the floor and straighten your legs as much as possible in front of you. Keep your back straight and lean slowly forward until you feel the stretch. Hold for 10 to 20 seconds. Return to the starting position. Repeat four to five times.

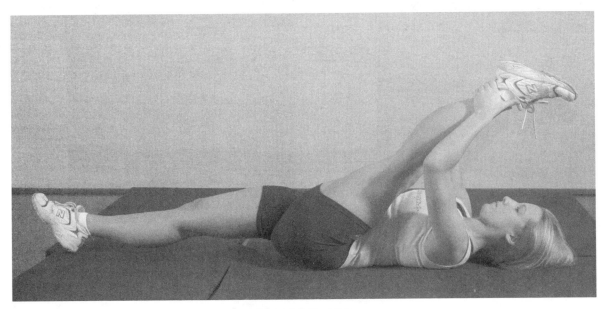

Hamstring Stretch 2

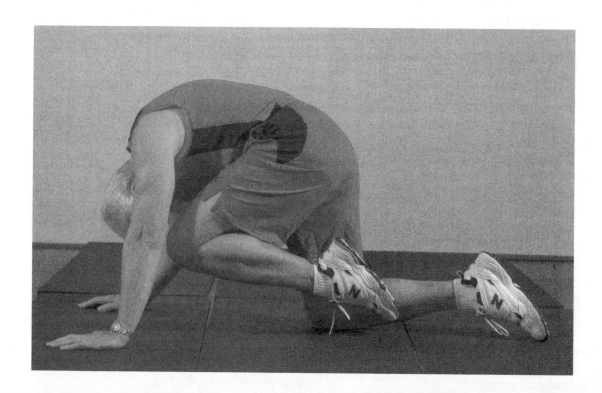

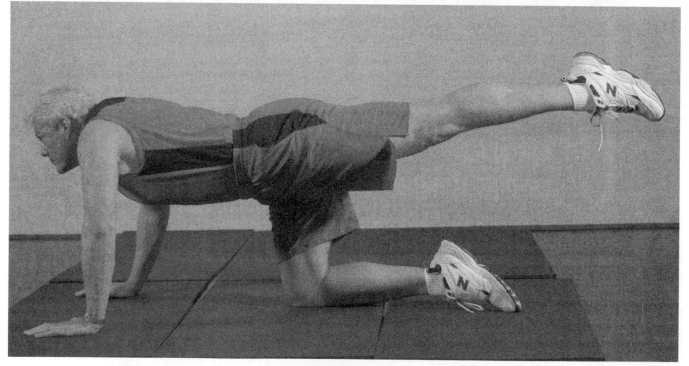

Leg Swoops

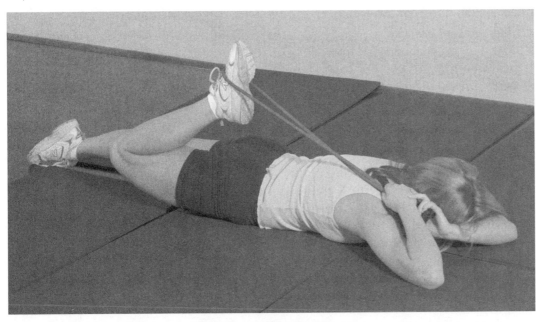

Quadriceps and Hamstring Stretch

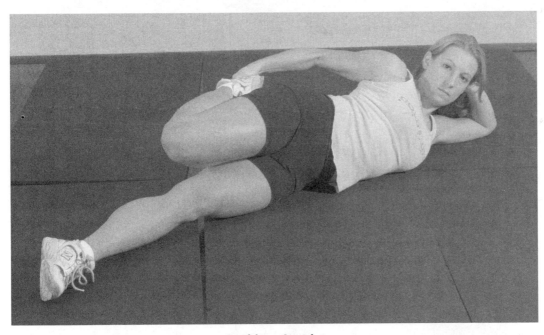

Quadriceps Stretch 1

Supine Hamstring Stretch

Lie on your back on the floor near a wall, with your buttocks toward the wall. Place one leg on the wall, pressing the leg against the wall with your foot and lower leg. Hold for 30 seconds. Relax. Slide your buttocks closer to the wall and repeat the exercise. Continue moving until your buttocks are as close to the wall as possible. Do three sets of 10. Repeat the exercise with the other leg.

Knee, Ankle, and Foot Stretches
Achilles Tendon Stretches

1. Stand an arm's length from a wall, and lean forward on your hands. Move one foot forward, and one foot slightly back. Keep the heel of the back foot flat on the floor. Stretch forward until you feel the stretch in the back of the knee. Hold for 10 seconds. Unlock the back knee and bend it toward the wall until you feel the stretch in the lower leg, closer to the heel. Hold for 10 seconds. Repeat eight to 10 times. Repeat the exercise with your other leg.

2. Kneel on the floor. Inhale as you shift one foot slightly forward. Keep the foot flat, with the bottom of the foot facing up. Exhale and lean forward. You will feel the stretch in the top of your foot. Hold the stretch, then relax. Repeat 10 times. Repeat the exercise with your other foot.

Ankle and Calf Stretch
Sit back in a chair, with your feet flat on the floor. Keeping your heels on the floor, lean forward in the chair. If necessary, push your knees down. Hold

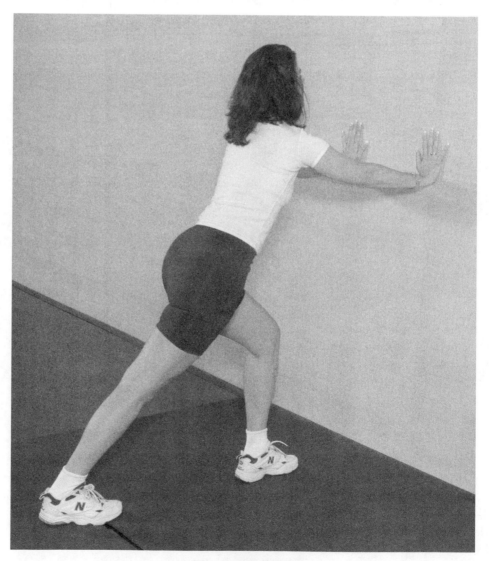

Achilles Tendon Stretch 1

for 45 seconds. Return to the starting position. Repeat five to 10 times.

Ankle Circles

Remove your shoes and socks. Sit on the floor or in a chair. Moving only your ankle, draw circles. Repeat 10 to 20 times. Repeat the exercise with your other ankle.

Ankle Tilt

Stand next to a support such as a counter or table, with your feet shoulder width apart. Holding onto the support, slowly bend and rotate your knees laterally and downward until you are standing on the outside of your ankles. Hold for 10 seconds. Slowly rotate your knees in the other direction until you are standing on the inside of your ankles. Repeat 10 to 20 times.

Ankle Stretch: Drawing the Alphabet

Remove your shoes and socks. Sit on the floor or in a chair. Moving only your ankle, draw the alphabet on the floor. Do the entire alphabet once. Repeat the exercise with your other ankle.

7

Weight Training: The Basics

Mention weight lifting, and some people have an image of hard-core bodybuilders with outsized biceps and no neck. But mention resistance training, and you won't get the same reaction. This is interesting, since a lot of resistance training involves moving weights. Think of resistance training as weight lifting without the cultural baggage.

There are many types of exercises that use resistance. The resistance may take the form of objects that you move, such as weights; stationary objects, such as a wall or the floor; or the weight of your own body. This chapter explains the basic principles of training with weights, which is a key part of a fitness program.

Weight training will increase the size and strength of your muscles. Or will it? If you go to the gym once in a while and pump some iron, you may feel good about it afterward (and probably be sore the next day), but if you don't follow a consistent routine, you won't achieve the long-term gains you're seeking. In addition, the actual act of lifting weights requires concentration

on technique, both to avoid injury and to get the maximum benefit from the exercise.

Go to any gym and you'll see all sorts of people lifting all types of weights. The people may be old or young, short or tall, heavy or thin, novice or expert, and so on. Your first assignment: Ignore them! Everyone brings his or her own unique experiences, goals, medical history, and body type to a training program. Your medical history and body type may be more important than your experiences and goals, particularly if you are just starting out. This is why individualization is crucial to any weight program: The guy pumping iron on the machine next to you may be an experienced weight lifter who can handle numerous repetitions at high intensity. Or he may be no more experienced than you are, but is trying to do too much, too fast—in which case he'll likely wind up with an injury. In either case, you should focus exclusively on your own program and what you're trying to accomplish.

Before beginning a weight training program, it is important to get a physical examination if you are over 35 years of age or have a preexisting condition or injury that may have an effect on the routine you choose. You need to tell your fitness trainer or instructor about any injuries you have had that might preclude you from performing certain exercises. For example, people with lower back problems should not perform squats. If you are rehabilitating an injury, it is absolutely imperative that you get the advice of your doctor or physical therapist before attempting any weight exercises.

The next order of business is to set goals for yourself. You probably have a general goal of "getting in shape" or improving your fitness, but what is it that you truly seek? Do you want to become stronger, and, if so, is it more important to increase your strength in your upper or lower body, or in specific muscle groups? Do you want to increase your muscle size? Do you want to improve your muscle endurance? Do you want to train with an eye toward improving your performance in a specific sport? The answers to these questions will determine what kind of program you develop with your trainer or instructor.

This process of training your body so it adapts in a specific way is called **specificity**. Training with weights is one part of developing a fit body, but your training routine should also include exercises that improve your flexibility and cardiovascular fitness. If you are an avid skier, for example, you might want to do exercises that increase your lower body strength and flexibility. Adding specificity to your training will help you achieve your goals more quickly.

Training with weights does not just involve lifting as much as you can for as long as you can. The way to build muscle strength and endurance without getting burned out is to vary the types of exercises, the intensity (the amount of weight), and the frequency. In general, more repetitions with lighter weights increase muscle endurance, while fewer repetitions with heavier weights increase power. Dynamic muscle actions (moving a weight through a range of motion) and isometric muscle actions (pushing against a stationary object) have different effects. With dynamic muscle actions, there is a concentric action (what you do when you raise a weight) and an eccentric action (when you lower it back down), and they have different effects too. Have your trainer or instructor match up your goals with the right types of exercises.

The process of lifting weights to make your muscles stronger is called **overloading**, and it's the basic principle of training with weights. When you lift weights, you are overloading your muscles and asking them to do more than they are used to doing. This forces them to adapt to the new stress.

If your muscle size and strength could increase merely through the normal, everyday activities of life, there would be a lot of people walking around with Mr./Ms. Universe–type bodies. Of course, that's not the case. It's also not the case that you can lift the same amount of weight the same number of times and continue to make fitness gains. Instead, you have to keep overloading your muscles once they adapt to a new level. This doesn't mean that you will keep lifting until you're bench-pressing 400 pounds, but it does mean that you will need to increase either the load (the amount of weight) or the sets and repetitions (the number of times you lift the weight) to make progress. This is done gradually, over a period of weeks, to lower the risk of injury from too much stress on your muscles and joints.

The key is to continually challenge your body without pushing it too far. For example, if you can comfortably do three sets of 10 repetitions at 100 pounds on a bench press, you can overload your muscles—and increase your strength—by adding an extra set or by lifting more weight but doing three sets of seven repetitions instead.

Variation is important in any overall fitness program, and this applies especially to the weight training part of your routine. Your trainer or instructor will give suggestions for substituting some exercises for others, as well as modifying the way you do certain exercises. The object of variation is to prevent you from getting burned out or hitting a plateau in your workouts.

There are many ways to vary your workouts. They can be as minor as changing the way you grip a barbell in a certain exercise, or as major as adding an entirely new set of exercises to your workout. You can also increase or decrease weight, repetitions, and rest time to add variety.

Rest is what you do when you're not working out—but this doesn't mean that your body is doing nothing. Between workouts, your body is recovering from the stresses you have placed on it. It is also adapting to those stresses so that it can bounce back even stronger for the next workout. Most of the changes your body undergoes during a training program take place not during the four or five hours you work out each week, but during the other 160-plus hours. Physically and psychologically, you *feel* your muscles working hard during a workout, but the real changes are taking place deeper down, at the neurological and cellular levels.

Frequency, or how often you should train, is dictated by a number of variables, among them your general conditioning level, your training goals, what point you have reached in your program, what type of exercises you are performing, and what intensity you are performing them at. Too infrequent

training will not enable you to reach your goals; too frequent training can leave you burned out or injured.

In general, it is recommended that you train on alternate days to allow your muscles adequate time to adapt to the new stresses on them; this is the schedule used in the sample programs described in this book. If you are well trained and have previous experience in resistance training programs, you may benefit from more-frequent workouts. For athletes just beginning a weight training program, however, it is very important to get adequate rest between workouts.

You may find that some muscles recover more quickly than others. In addition, muscles take longer to recover from multiple-joint exercises, which place stress on more than one joint (Squats using a barbell, for instance), than they do from single-joint exercises like Biceps Curls and Knee Extensions.

If you are recovering from an injury or illness, you should return gradually to your previous level of workout frequency. If you were going to the gym three times a week and then missed two weeks due to illness, a business trip, or one of life's other unavoidable interruptions, you should probably not resume your program with three workout days the week you return. Always err on the side of caution when dealing with injuries or illness.

On a macro level, it is recommended that you take at least 24 hours off between workouts to let your body rest and adapt. Make good use of the time before your next workout by eating a balanced diet (see Chapter 11 on nutrition) and getting enough sleep. These lifestyle elements are as important as what you do in the gym or on the playing field.

On a micro level, the rest periods between sets and between exercises will vary according to the type of program you are following. For example, a high-intensity exercise that is performed for 30 seconds may require up to three minutes for your body to replenish the phosphagen stores in your muscles.

You may benefit from longer rest periods between sets. This is especially true for heavier athletes, as well as for those who are just beginning a weight training program. Some coaches and athletes make sure that the heart rate returns to a certain level before beginning the next set. Consult your coach or trainer if you are unsure about how much rest to take between sets at any given point in your program.

How much rest is too much? There is a limit to how much time you rest before you start to lose the fitness gains you've made. This is called "detraining." Fortunately, studies have shown that taking a week off—even two, in some cases—may not cause a significant loss in conditioning. This assumes, of course, that you've already reached a certain level of fitness and aren't just starting out. The benefit is that if you have been pushing yourself in the weeks preceding a break, the time off will allow your body to rejuvenate itself, leaving you refreshed and ready when you resume workouts.

TYPES OF RESISTANCE

With the recent proliferation of fitness gadgets and machines—ThighMaster, anyone?—it can be confusing to figure out which ones work and which ones best suit your needs. The following sections describe the basic types of resistance training equipment you're likely to find at most gyms. (Chapter 12 offers detailed descriptions of the different types of machines available for home use. Before using any of them, be sure to learn the proper technique from qualified trainers or gym personnel.)

Weight Machines and Free Weights: Which Is Better?

If you're just beginning to lift weights or if you haven't done any weight training for a long time, it's important to consider the advantages and disadvantages of weight machines and free weights. Both can help you achieve your fitness goals, but they do so in different ways.

A weight machine is a stationary apparatus that uses a system of pulleys or pistons to provide resistance. Free weights consist of dumbbells and barbells to which you add weighted plates.

For most beginners, weight machines are the preferred method of training, although you will notice that some of the exercises described later in this book use dumbbells. Dumbbells are useful for beginners because they offer the wide range of motion of free weights, but with little risk of injury, since they are easier to balance than barbells.

Here are some advantages of weight machines:

- Weight machines are easy to use: You insert a pin into a stack of weights and you're ready to exercise. You can easily add or subtract weight for a particular exercise.
- Weight machines don't require as much concentration on technique as free weights do; they give you greater control over the weight as you are moving it. This lessens (but does not eliminate) the risk of injury.
- Different types of weight machines offer different types of resistance, so you often have several options to choose from at the same gym.

And here are some disadvantages of weight machines:

- Weight machines offer a limited number of exercises and a limited range of motion within each exercise, compared to free weights. This means that your muscles may not be getting the maximum benefit from some exercises if you're performing them on a weight machine instead of using free weights.

- Weight machines are more expensive to purchase and maintain than free weights. This is important if you're interested in setting up a gym or workout room in your home. (See Chapter 12 on buying home exercise equipment.)

Here are some advantages of free weights:

- Free weights allow you to use a greater range of motion than weight machines.
- Free weights force you to coordinate several muscle groups to perform each exercise, which gives you a greater overall benefit.
- Free weights are cheaper to purchase and easier to maintain than weight machines.

And here are some disadvantages of free weights:

- Free weights offer less control over the weight, which increases your risk of injury.
- Free weights require more training in technique than weight machines, because you have to learn how to use some muscles as stabilizers during each exercise in order to keep the weight under control. Many exercises require a spotter (someone to assist the weight lifter in difficult exercises or those involving heavy weights).
- Loose weights, barbells, and dumbbells lying around can create an unsafe workout environment.

Other Types of Resistance

In the past few decades, there has been an explosion of fitness equipment using forms of resistance that don't involve traditional weights. Most of this equipment won't give you bulging biceps or massive pecs—such muscle transformations are usually achieved only with the use of free weights over an extended period of time. But this equipment can be effective in toning muscles and giving you a fitter-looking body.

Before you start using a machine or device that works on one of the principles listed below, talk to your personal trainer or gym personnel about how it works and whether it's going to help you achieve your goals.

- Machines like stationary cycles and some wrist-curl devices use **friction** to provide resistance. With these machines, you generally expend more energy initially and then maintain a constant level to continue the exercise.
- Machines that use cylinders and pistons provide **fluid resistance** and are good at simulating the kind of resistance encountered in sports like running and swimming. You'll often find that as you move through an exercise on one of these machines, the resistance increases, so that if you are doing a bench press, for instance, it feels as though you're working harder the closer you get to the top of the lift. The emphasis here is on the concentric, rather than the eccentric, action.
- **Elasticity** is a form of resistance used in many home gym units that employ a system of springs or heavy rubber bands. These exercises provide low resistance at the beginning of the motion and high resistance toward the end. This can be problematic, because your muscles work in the opposite manner, that is, they are capable of exerting more force at the beginning of a range of motion and less at the end.

SAFETY WITH WEIGHTS

It is easy to injure yourself when you're lifting weights, and not just by dropping a 20-pound dumbbell on your foot. The reason for this is fairly simple: Unlike activities such as running, cycling, or playing sports, when you lift weights, you are putting excessive stress on one muscle or group of muscles. You might, in fact, put more concentrated, continuous strain on your quadriceps during three sets of leg lifts than you would during a full-court basketball game.

It is very important, then, to be smart when you are lifting weights, particularly if you are doing it for the first time or haven't done it for some time. You should expect some degree of muscle soreness, especially in the first several weeks of workouts (and soreness is usually a good sign). However, if you push your muscles too hard or ask them to do things they're not capable of doing, they will rebel by straining, pulling, or tearing (and these are always a bad sign). There are few things more frustrating than establishing a good workout routine and then suddenly having to suspend it for days or weeks while you rehabilitate an injury that could have been avoided with better preparation or technique.

Technique

In every one of life's activities, there is no substitute for good technique. In the gym, it can be the difference between a vigorous, satisfying workout and one that leaves you nursing a muscle pull and looking forward to two weeks on the shelf.

Correct technique will decrease your risk of injury; it will also tell your muscles how to properly respond to specific exercises. A slight difference in the angle of your back or knees or head, for example, can determine whether you will get the maximum benefit from an exercise. Unfortunately, many people do not know the correct technique for even the most familiar exercises, which is why it is important to get proper instruction from a qualified trainer or instructor. The pictures and descriptions included in this book should be used as a guide, but you should not attempt an exercise using weights for the first time without being supervised by a professional trainer.

Muscle Imbalances: An Argument for Cross-Training

It's great if you specialize in one thing and do it really well. But with fitness training, such specialization can create muscle imbalances that leave you at risk of injury and unprepared for doing other types of exercises. Athletes who play one sport year-round, for instance, may be strengthening some muscle groups at the expense of others.

Cross-training is a word that has been in vogue for some time, and it simply means including different types of activities in your training program. Presumably, you are already doing this as part of your weekly workout routine. But it is useful to remember that varying your exercise activities not only keeps you motivated and fresh—it gets your muscles and joints working in a variety of ways. If you are starting a conditioning program, cross-training means varying the aerobic part of your routine to include activities like biking, swimming, and jogging and using machines like elliptical trainers and stair-climbers. All of these will get your heart pumping, but they also place different stresses on your muscles and joints.

Safety Tips

Here are some general safety tips for training with weights:

- Never attempt a weight exercise without first learning the technique under the supervision of qualified gym personnel. The majority of weight training injuries are caused by improper technique, and they often occur in the home, where there is no supervision. Learn it, practice it, then perform it.

- Warm up and stretch before you work out. It is surprising how many people neglect to perform these basic prevention techniques. You are about to ask your muscles to take on unnatural stress, so it makes sense to make sure they are warm and limber and ready for the stress.

- Before you lift weights, it is sometimes useful to do a warm-up set of each exercise. This consists of one set at about 50 percent of the weight you will be lifting in the full exercise. Ask your trainer for advice in this regard.

- Perform all exercise with a controlled, fluid motion. Don't rush, and don't use a jerky motion. If it takes a jerky, awkward motion to lift a particular weight, it means that you're attempting to lift too much and should decrease the weight.

- Breathe! This sounds easy, yet it is amazing how many people try to lift weights while holding their breath. A good rule to follow is to exhale on the initial thrust of the exercise (pushing the bar upward, for example) and inhale on the second part of the motion.

- "Start fast, end slow." In general, you want to take about half as long to raise the weight as you do to bring it down. The first part of the motion is the concentric motion, in which your muscles shorten. The second part is the eccentric motion, in which your muscles lengthen. Performing the second part of the motion slowly will increase the benefit to your muscles.

- If you are using a dumbbell or barbell, keep the weight close to your body. The farther away it is, the less control you have—and the greater the chance that you will suffer an injury.

- If you must turn while lifting a weight, turn your whole body instead of just your lower back or hips. This will reduce stress on those areas.

- Bend your knees slightly when you are performing dumbbell or barbell exercises from a standing position. This will reduce pressure on your lower back.

- Keep your back as straight as possible when you are doing weight exercises. If it is curved or arched, you are forcing it to take on too much stress.

- When doing exercises from a standing position, spread your chest and keep your shoulders back, not rounded.

- To decrease the risk of injury to your shoulders, make sure that you are warmed up and have performed stretching exercises to loosen up your shoulder area. Above all, use proper technique when doing exercises like Bench Presses and Lat Pulls, which place a great deal of stress on your shoulders.

- If you are learning a new exercise or have been away from training for a week or two, always begin with lighter weight than you will eventually be lifting. This will get your muscles and joints used to the new motion without forcing them to withstand too much stress.

SAFETY AT THE GYM

With more and more people taking part in weight training, the number of related injuries is rising. As noted above, the majority of these injuries result from improper technique and lack of proper supervision. This does not mean, however, that the majority of these injuries occur in the home. The gym environment, while providing the machines and apparatus necessary for a workout, can be as treacherous as its counterpart in the home.

The following list of safety measures is adapted from guidelines formulated by the National Strength and Conditioning Association (NSCA):

- Exercise machines should be assembled and tested by professionals before they are used in training programs.
- There should be 100 square feet of training space for every person using an area at any one time, depending on the type of equipment being used.
- Equipment must be regularly inspected and maintained, with inspection records kept. Damaged equipment should not be used; it should be removed from use until repaired.
- All equipment should be cleaned and/or disinfected regularly, and athletes should be encouraged to wipe down skin-contact surfaces after use.
- Signs describing appropriate use and including warnings should be posted for all equipment.
- Strength and conditioning supervisors should have a bachelor's or master's degree from an accredited college or university.
- Supervisors must have CPR and blood-borne pathogen training.
- Supervisors must be present during all activities, with a clear view of all participants, and close enough to provide assistance or spotting when needed.
- An emergency response plan should be developed, posted, and rehearsed. An emergency telephone should be readily accessible at all times.
- Strength and conditioning professionals must not prescribe, recommend, or provide drugs, controlled substances, or supplements that are illegal, prohibited, or harmful to athletes for any purpose, including enhancing athletic performance, conditioning, or physique.

8

Specific Training Programs

This chapter provides examples of workout routines that you can use to achieve a basic level of fitness, separated into men's and women's beginner and intermediate workouts. Since everyone brings to training a unique combination of fitness level and relevant injuries and medical conditions, these programs should be used as a basis from which you can develop your own routine.

You will notice that the programs include a full range of activities: warm-up, stretching, exercises with weights, aerobic exercise, and cool-down. Some of the exercises may be easy for you to do; others may not. If you cannot perform some exercises as described, find a variation that will achieve the same purpose.

THE EXERCISES

Some of the exercises in this section involve weights, and some do not. Exercises that use only the resistance of your own body weight may be most effective, because they are specific to you. With all exercises, and particularly with those that involve weights, pay attention to technique and to the need for rest. If you are fatigued, form is the first thing you lose—and that can lead to injury. Rest! Particularly in the first few weeks, you may find yourself out of breath frequently. Slow down and let your heart rate decrease before moving on to the next exercise.

There is logic in the order of the exercises presented. For example, Leg Extension is followed by Leg Press: Even though you are working the same body area, you are using opposing motions. Each workout also proceeds from focusing on your largest muscle group to your smallest, since exercises for larger muscles pre-fatigue the smaller muscle groups. Thus, after you have done lunges, your quads are ready to do leg extensions.

BREATHING AND FOCUSING

Concentrate on breathing during each exercise. Breathe out during contraction—when you are pushing a weight upward, for instance—and breathe in during relaxation. As you perform each exercise, it may be helpful if you paint a mental image of what your muscles have to do, then put that image into action.

In order to get the maximum benefit from an exercise, concentrate on the motion and contraction of the particular muscle or muscle group being exercised. A common error is overgripping a barbell or dumbbell, which can place stress on the fingers, wrists, and forearms instead of on the muscle(s) targeted by the exercise.

One of the keys to successful training (and to almost every other pursuit, as well) is being able to focus on exactly what you are about to do, and nothing else. The ability to focus is particularly helpful when you're doing several exercises in succession that overload different muscle groups.

There can be a lot of distractions at the gym: music, televisions playing in the background, people and machines in constant (and sometimes noisy) motion. Remember that this is *your* workout, not the workout of the person next to you or your friend or the hottie on the exercise bike whose eye you're trying to catch. Concentrate on what *you* have to do. If you're looking for a partner, you may be better off at a singles bar than a gym.

TECHNIQUE: DOING IT RIGHT

Never perform a new exercise without first learning the proper technique under the supervision of qualified gym personnel. Although the techniques described in many of the exercises below may seem self-explanatory—push-ups and pull-ups, for example—all of them can cause unnecessary soreness or injury if not performed with the proper technique. The time

to learn how to do something the right way is always time well spent.

Have you ever noticed all the mirrors in a gym? Did you assume that their purpose is to allow people to admire their rippling muscles? Think again! The best way to make sure you are using the correct form is to watch yourself in a mirror. For example, even though you think you are performing an exercise correctly, you may notice in the mirror that the angle of your arms is slightly off or that you are holding your head in the wrong position. This is especially true for exercises that require you to keep your back straight and not arched. Mirrors allow you to take a peek and see for yourself.

KEEPING A WORKOUT LOG

You can use a workout log supplied by the gym, or you can make your own by putting copies of your exercise list in a loose-leaf binder—or in a small spiral notebook that fits in your pocket. By keeping a log, you will have a record of your progress and can make changes to your routine based on how you are doing. Be faithful; follow the instructions in the program and use the log. Write comments about specific exercises. If you have a problem with or question about a certain exercise, the log is the place to write it down.

MEASURING THE HEART RATE

As noted earlier in this book, it is important to check your heart rate before, during, and after your workout. Before you start your warm-up, record your heart rate in your log. At the end of your workout, wait about 15 minutes before you check your heart rate. This is your recovery rate, a measure of how fast your heart returns to its normal rate. Your recovery rate should be about your normal resting heart rate.

If you are beginning a workout routine for the first time, you may have a resting heart rate of about 90 beats per minute. In the middle of your workout, that number should reach about 120. Fifteen minutes after the end of your workout, your rate should be about 80. Over time, you should notice that your heart rate is dropping the more you work out. Your resting heart rate will decrease after several weeks; this is a sign that your cardiovascular system is learning to adapt as you continue your training.

If your heart rate is too low or too high, you need to stop exercising. Your body is like a car engine: If it's idling too slowly, it may stall, and if it's idling too quickly, you may wind up with a "carburetor"—or other systemic—problem.

WARM-UP

Start each workout session with a moderate, six-minute warm-up. Walking on a treadmill or riding a stationary bike are excellent ways to warm up, in part because they make it easy for you to monitor yourself. Cross-trainers and other aerobic machines are fine as well, although a beginner may find them more complex than a treadmill or stationary bike. Remember: A warm-up is not a race. You should not be looking to raise your heart rate significantly. The goal is to get your blood flowing.

Another important step in your preparation is to think about what you will do in your workout. Imagine yourself performing each movement perfectly. Control your breathing by taking deep breaths. Think of your workout as something that you do for yourself, to make yourself feel better

and become more fit. This focused visualization is one of the most effective tools you can use in the early stages of fitness training. Elite, world-class athletes make this visualization a regular part of their workouts.

After you have completed your warm-up, check your heart rate and record it in your log.

STRETCHING

Your warm-up will have gotten the blood flowing to your muscles and prepared you for stretching. For a description of specific stretching exercises, see Chapter 6. You don't have to spend a lot of time stretching, but you should make sure to stretch your arms and shoulders, trunk, lower back, quadriceps, hamstrings, and calves. A few minutes of stretching at the beginning of your workout can prevent a lot of soreness the next day.

SAMPLE WORKOUTS

Women's Beginner Workout

This is a six-week beginner program for women. Follow the program exactly; when the six weeks is up, you will be able to make changes. In addition to overloading your muscles, you will be teaching them to work together correctly—which takes time. You are giving your body a chance to adapt to weight-bearing exercises. If you proceed gradually, you won't experience undue soreness. Remember that some soreness is normal on the day after a workout, because your body is adapting to new stresses.

Rest between exercises for a minute or two, or however long it takes to move from one machine to another. Don't hurry—but don't dawdle either, or your muscles will get cold and you will lose your momentum.

Single Stationary Lunge

This is one of the most effective exercises for the upper thigh and glute area. You'll feel the contraction in your lower quadriceps the most. After the exercise, be sure to stretch your quadriceps.

Body areas affected: Quadriceps, glutes, and hamstrings.

Equipment needed: Floor mat or any soft, flat surface.

Weight: Body weight.

Technique: Stand erect with your feet shoulder-width apart. Take one full step forward with your right leg so that your right foot is two feet in front of your left. Your weight should be evenly distributed. Lift your left heel, and move your left hip forward slightly into a pelvic tilt so that your left thigh is perpendicular to the floor. Hold that position, then slowly lower yourself until your left knee nearly touches the floor. Your lower body should be in contraction, including your abdomen, hamstrings, and quads. As you rise, concentrate on squeezing your legs together. Keep your feet in position.

Sets and reps: Do 15 reps with your right leg forward, then 15 with your left leg forward.

Tips: Exhale while moving downward, and inhale on the way up. *Go slowly!* Each rep should take about 10 seconds to complete. Count "one-

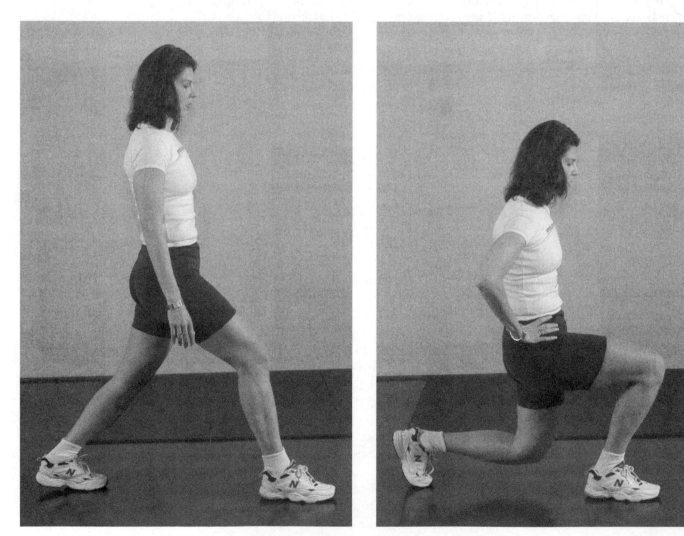

Single Stationary Lunge

one-thousand, two-one-thousand," and so on. Take four seconds for the positive motion (moving downward) and 6 seconds for the negative (rising). Concentrate on holding the contraction and squeezing the muscles. If you need assistance in balancing, steady yourself with a chair or a wall.

Calf Raise

This exercise might seem easy to do—almost too easy—but overdoing it can have painful results. Go slowly. Remember that you are building a foundation for more challenging workouts.

Body areas affected: Feet, calves, and ankles.

Equipment needed: Stair step or other raised platform.

Weight: Body weight.

Technique: Stand on the platform with your feet together and your heels slightly over the edge. Allow your heels to fall. Feel the stretch in your lower legs. Control the stretch and hold it. Slowly raise your heels up, contracting your calves, and lift yourself on your tiptoes so that your heels are as high as possible. Come to full contraction at the top of the exercise and fully stretch your calves with each repetition.

Calf Raise

Sets and reps: One set of 12 to 15 repetitions, using both legs at once. If you feel you are able to add another set after three weeks, do so.

Tip: The idea is not to just move your heels up and down. Start by contracting your big toe, and then contract the entire foot.

Upright Row

Body areas affected: Deltoids, upper back, trapezoids, and scapulas.

Equipment needed: Light barbell or dumbbells.

Weight: Three-, five-, or eight-pound dumbbells, depending on what feels comfortable to you, or a very light barbell.

Technique: If you are using dumbbells, hold them in front of you, using an overhand grip and keeping your hands close together. If you are using a barbell, hold it in front of you, using an overhand grip and with your hands

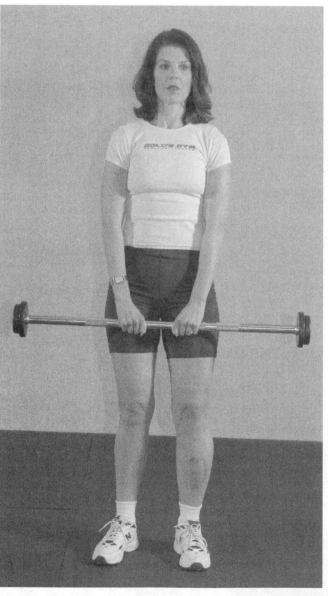 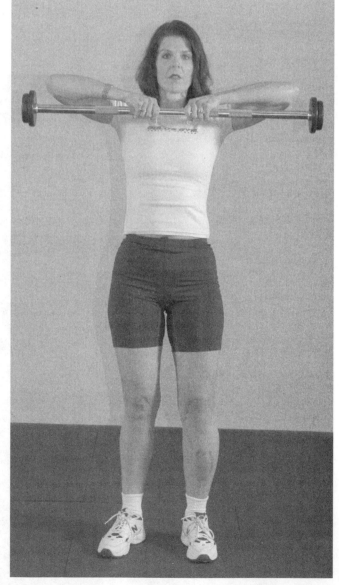

Upright Row

close enough together so that your thumbs would touch if you extended them. Standing erect with your feet shoulder-width apart and with your knees slightly bent, exhale and pull the bar or dumbbells up near your body (parallel to your trunk) to about an inch below your chin. Hold for a second, then relax and slowly lower the weight.

Sets and reps: Two sets of 10 to 12 repetitions.

Tip: Relax your hands! Overgripping is the cause of many injuries.

Push-Ups

Body areas affected: Chest, biceps, and triceps.

Equipment needed: Floor mat or flat, nonslippery surface.

Weight: Body weight.

Technique: Get into the standard push-up position, raised up on your arms with your legs extended and your feet together. Try not to lock your arms in this position. Slowly lower yourself until your nose is nearly touching the floor. Raise yourself back up by pushing with your arms. Keep your back flat throughout the exercise.

Sets and reps: Start with five push-ups, and each day try to do at least one more. If you get up to 15, try to do two sets of 10.

Tips: Go slowly—this will help you get the full benefit of the exercise. If you must do this exercise with your knees on the floor in the beginning, that's okay, but gradually try to do the push-ups with your legs extended.

Chest Flye (illustrated on p. 64)

Body areas affected: Chest and biceps.

Equipment needed: Weight bench or other flat bench; light dumbbells.

Weight: Three-, five-, or eight-pound dumbbells, depending on what feels comfortable to you.

Technique: Lie on your back on the bench with your arms perpendicular to your body and slightly bowed (not locked at the elbow). Slowly bring the dumbbells together over your chest, then slowly back to the starting position. Force your lower back into the bench at all times—don't arch it. Hold the contraction during each rep of this exercise. Concentrate on balancing the weights and keeping them even.

Sets and reps: Two sets of 8 to 10 repetitions.

Tip: To keep your back flat on the bench, it's best to bend your knees and keep your feet on the bench.

Front Raise (illustrated on p. 65)

Body areas affected: Shoulders, triceps, and deltoids.

Equipment needed: Light dumbbells.

Weight: Three-, five-, or eight-pound dumbbells, depending on what feels comfortable to you.

Technique: Hold the dumbbells as you would for the Upright Row, with an overhand grip and with the weights resting against your thighs. Slowly raise a dumbbell straight out in front of you until your arm is parallel to the floor, then lower it back to the starting position.

Sets and reps: Two sets of 10 to 12 repetitions.

Tip: You can do this exercise with both arms at the same time, but it's probably best to alternate arms when you are starting out.

Biceps Curl (illustrated on p. 66)

Body area affected: Upper arms.

Equipment needed: Light dumbbells.

Weight: Three-, five-, or eight-pound dumbbells, depending on what feels comfortable to you.

Technique: Stand erect with your feet shoulder-width apart. Hold the

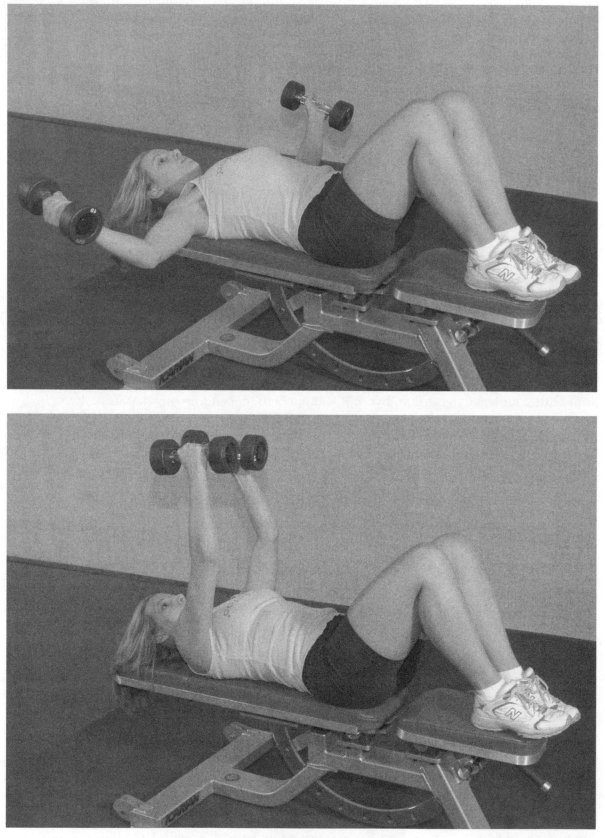

Chest Flye

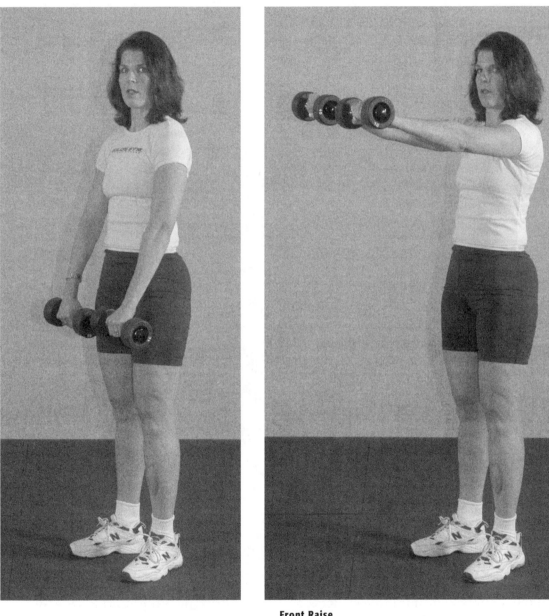

Front Raise

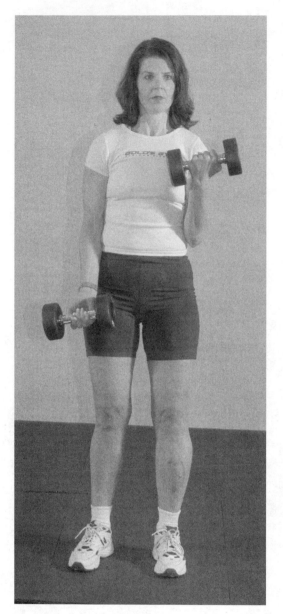
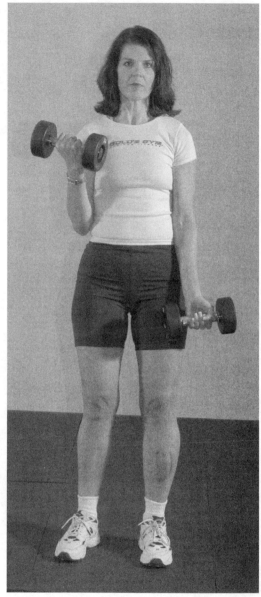

Biceps Curl

dumbbells with an underhand grip and let them rest against your thighs. Flex your left arm at the elbow, raise the dumbbell until it is a few inches from your chest, then lower it to the starting position. Repeat with your right arm. Go slowly, and continue to concentrate on your breathing.

Sets and reps: Two sets of 10 repetitions, alternating arms (10 left, 10 right, 10 left, 10 right). Alternating arms at each repetition wouldn't cause enough muscle fatigue in the arm.

Tips: The Biceps Curl looks easy to do but is often done incorrectly. To make sure that you are isolating your biceps, start the motion with your upper arms flush against your ribs. Keep your elbows and upper arm stationary through the entire motion.

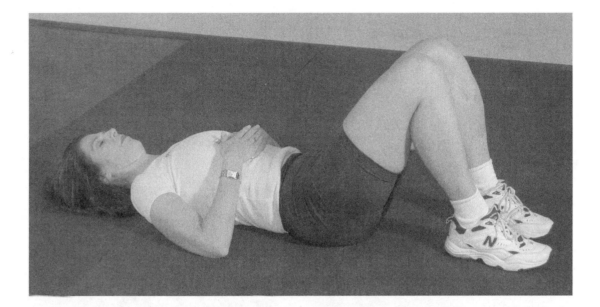

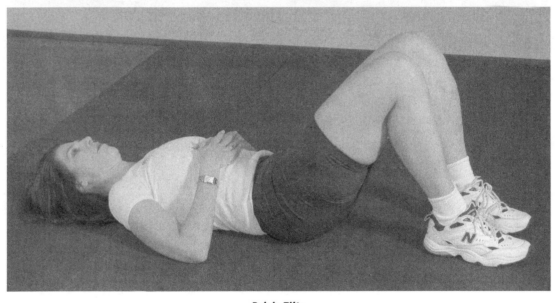

Pelvic Tilts

Pelvic Tilts

Body area affected: Lower back.

Equipment needed: Workout mat or flat, nonslippery surface.

Weight: Body weight.

Technique: Lie on your back with your knees bent and your feet flat on the floor. Slowly contract your lower abdomen and lower back by pressing your lower back into the floor and squeezing your buttocks together.

Your hips should remain flat on the floor.

Sets and reps: Two sets of 15 repetitions.

Crunches (illustrated on p. 68)

Body areas affected: Trunk and abdominals.

Equipment needed: Workout mat or flat, nonslippery surface.

Weight: Body weight.

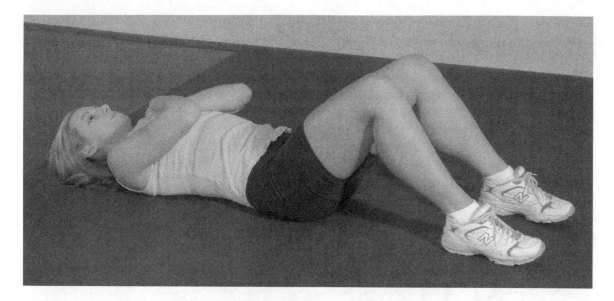

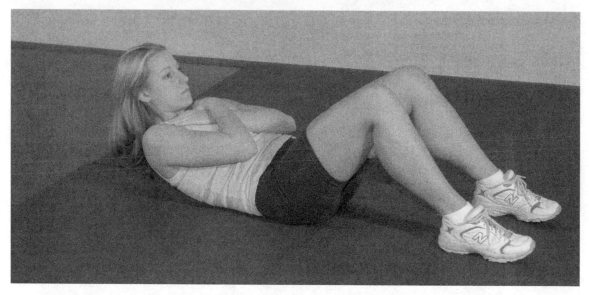

Crunches

Technique: Lie on your back with your legs bent and your feet flat on the floor. Clasp your hands across your chest and slowly curl your trunk upward by raising your chest and shoulders off the floor. Keep your lower back flat on the floor.

Sets and reps: Two sets of 10 to 15 repetitions.

Tips: Go slowly. Take four seconds to lift up and four seconds to lower your chest and shoulders back down. Once you have mastered this exercise, you can make it more challenging by holding a weight plate on your chest as you raise and lower.

Posture Awareness Exercise

Body areas affected: Lower back, abdominals, trunk, neck, and shoulders.

Equipment needed: Workout mat or flat, nonslippery surface.

Weight: Body weight.

Technique: Lie on your back on the floor with your legs and arms extended, and stretch yourself as long as you can.

Let your body relax. Slowly press your lower back into the floor for a count of four; do this 10 times, imagining that your back is melting into the floor. Stretch long again for a count of four; do this 10 times. Pull your knees toward your chest and move your nose toward your knees, rolling yourself into a ball. Keep your back on the floor and don't arch it. Exhale and relax into an extended position again. When you do the stretch the first few times, you may feel a slight headache; this is the result of stretching muscles in your neck and head that are not used to being stretched.

Cardiovascular Workout

Finish your workout with an aerobic activity. This can be done on a treadmill, stationary bike, elliptical trainer, stair-climber, or any machine that keeps you moving continuously and raises your heart rate. (You can also jog or ride a real bike, of course.) This is not a race; maintain a moderate pace and continue for 20 to 30 minutes. Check your heart rate halfway through and at the end of the exercise, recording both rates in your log. Check your heart rate a final time 15 minutes after you've finished your aerobic activity.

If you are embarking on a training program for the first time, these exercises may make you too tired to do the cardio workout. You may skip the cardio workout for the first workout or two, but in order to get a complete workout, you need to do the cardio workout.

The Finish

Don't stop abruptly when you have finished your workout. Do some light stretching and keep moving around for a few minutes to prevent the buildup of lactic acid in your muscles, which can cause muscle fatigue and cramping.

Women's Intermediate Workout

The intermediate workout includes new exercises, as well as some exercises from the beginner workout that increase the resistance weight. Proceed gradually when you add weight; if an exercise feels uncomfortable, go back to a lighter weight or no weight. Concentrate on form, balance, and isolating the correct muscles. If you have any questions, ask your trainer or qualified gym personnel.

Rest between exercises for a minute or two, or however long it takes to move from one machine to another. Don't hurry—but don't dawdle either, or your muscles will get cold and you will lose your momentum, both physically and psychologically.

Day 1: Legs, Back, Shoulders, and Arms

Weighted Stationary Lunge
For this exercise, you use the same motion as described in the Single Stationary Lunges in the beginner program, but you use dumbbells. Do two sets of 12 to 15 repetitions each. Hold the dumbbells loosely at your sides with an overhand grip.

Tips: Balance and posture are important in this exercise, particularly since you are now supporting extra weight. Form becomes especially important; make sure you have proper supervision for this exercise, particularly if you are using a barbell instead of dumbbells. Adding weight forces you to concentrate on balance, but it also helps to increase your strength more quickly.

Leg Extension (illustrated on pp. 70–71)
Body area affected: Quadriceps.
Equipment needed: Universal or Nautilus leg extension machine.
Weight: Use moderate weight to start, then gradually increase it in later workouts. If your quadriceps are sore

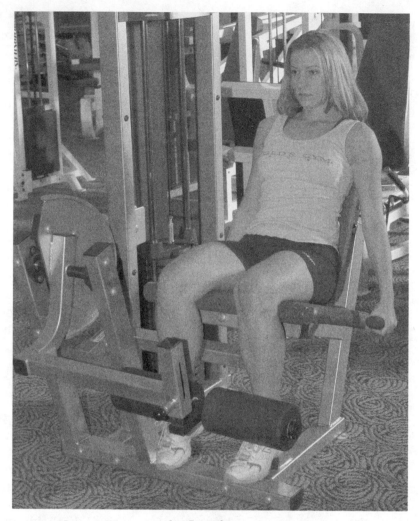

Leg Extension...

the next day, you probably set the weight too high. The tendency is to start with too heavy weight in this exercise.

Technique: Keep your back flush against the seat; use a seatbelt if one is available. Your knees should be off the edge of the seat. Lift the weight by extending your knees until they are fully extended at the top of the motion. Contract the muscle and hold for two seconds, then slowly return to the starting position.

Sets and reps: Two sets of 12 to 15 repetitions.

Tip: On the return motion, be sure to keep your feet in a flexed position with your toes up. If your toes are pointed, you will put undue pressure on your patellar tendon (the tendon in front of and below your kneecap).

Leg Press (illustrated on p. 72)
Leg Presses are similar to Squats, but they are more stable and less likely to injure your lower back, since you are sitting in a chair with back support.

Body areas affected: Lower legs and glutes.

Equipment needed: Universal or Nautilus leg press machine.

Weight: Light weight to start; you may add more gradually as you get used to the exercise.

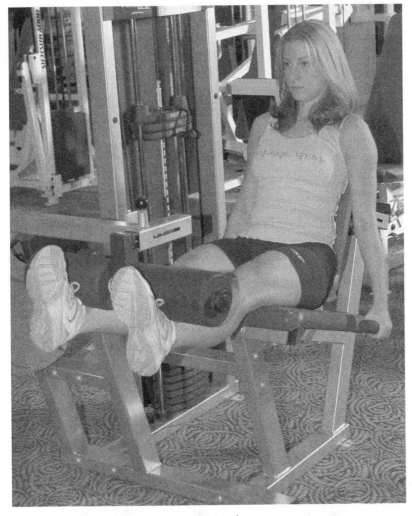

. . . Leg Extension

Technique: Sit in the chair and place your feet on the footpads. Keep your hips flat against the seat, and focus on going slowly. Starting with a light weight that you can comfortably handle, push against the weight until your legs are almost fully extended. Slowly return to the starting position by bending your knees.

Sets and reps: Two sets of 12 to 15 repetitions.

Tips: Have a trainer set up the chair correctly for your height and body type. When you do the eccentric (second) half of the motion, your feet should not be behind your knees, or you will place too much stress on your knees. Don't lock your knees at the top of the motion.

Calf Raise

Body areas affected: Calves and lower legs.

Equipment needed: Dumbbells or leg press machine.

Weight: Start with light weight (five- or 10-pound dumbbells or their equivalent).

Technique: Perform this exercise as in the beginner program, but using weight. Hold one dumbbell in each hand at your side. Alternatively, you can save time by using a leg press machine for this exercise. Push the

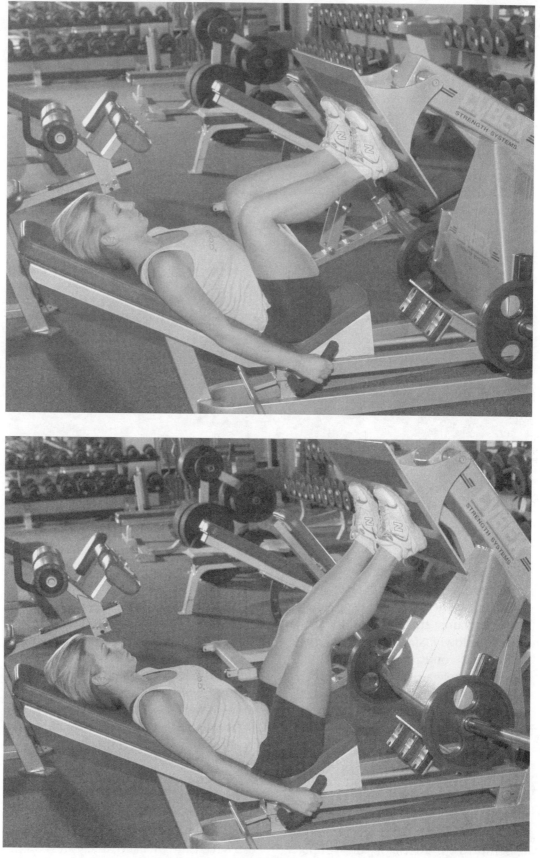

Leg Press

weight with your feet and then hold it there, sliding your feet down so that they are on the edge of the footpads, letting the weight come back slightly, then pushing it forward with the balls and toes of your feet.

Sets and reps: Two sets of 15 to 20 repetitions.

Tip: Be sure to take the weight off the machine before you do this for the first time. As you become more comfortable with the exercise, you can add weight gradually. Using too much weight when you are doing this exercise for the first time will almost guarantee sore calf muscles the next day.

Upright Row (illustrated on p. 62)

Follow the same form as described for the Upright Row in the beginner program, but add a little more weight. If you were using an eight-pound barbell before, go to 10 pounds, or go to the next heavier dumbbell.

Sets and reps: Two sets of 10 to 12 repetitions.

Lat Pulldown (illustrated on p. 74)

Body areas affected: Latissimus dorsi muscles (lats) and biceps.

Equipment needed: Lat machine.

Weight: Start with light weight initially, then increase weight gradually.

Technique: Depending on the height of the machine and the length of the pulley, you can do this exercise while sitting on a padded chair or kneeling with your feet crossed behind you. Drop your head forward and keep your back straight. Raise your arms and grab the bar above your head in an overhand grip; your hands can be close together—about eight inches apart—or you can grip the ends of the bar. Slowly pull the bar down toward the back of your neck, pulling with your shoulders and arms. To return to the starting position, slowly let the bar go back up—first with your arms, then with your shoulder blades. Alternatively, you can lean your head back and pull the weight down in front of your neck.

Sets and reps: Two sets of 10 to 12 repetitions.

Tip: Concentrate on pulling down with your shoulder blades first, as this forces your lats to do the work. If you pull the weight down with your arms, the primary muscle used will be the biceps.

Chest Flye (illustrated on p. 64)

Follow the form described for this exercise in the beginner program. Although you can use either a machine or dumbbells, a machine may be better, since it allows less variation in the motion. Increase the weight slightly from what you used in the beginner program.

Sets and reps: Two sets of 10 to 12 repetitions.

Tip: To get the maximum benefit from the exercise, bring your hands together above the middle of your chest, not above your neck or your waist.

Push-Ups

This is the same exercise as in the beginner program, but do only one set of as many repetitions as you can. Concentrate on good form as you begin to get fatigued. Go slowly.

Front Raise (illustrated on p. 65)

Follow the form described for this exercise in the beginner program, but increase the weight a little if it feels comfortable to you.

Sets and reps: Two sets of 10 to 12 repetitions.

Tips: The deltoid muscle is more difficult to build than other muscles because it is not used a lot. If you perform this exercise regularly, you will definitely add size to your deltoids.

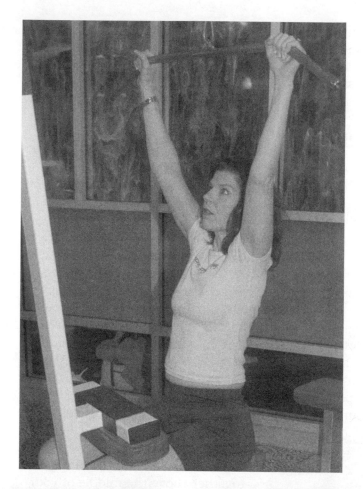

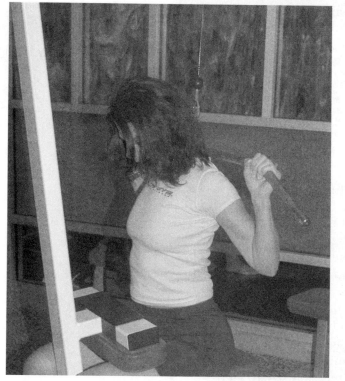

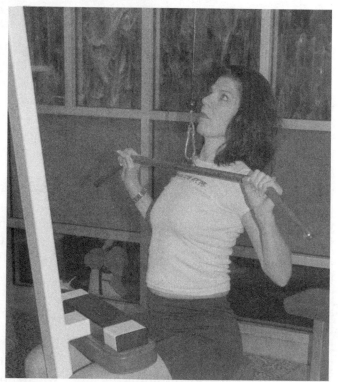

Lat Pulldown

Dumbbell Lateral Raise

Body area affected: Deltoids.

Equipment needed: Bench and dumbbells or Nautilus lateral raise machine.

Weight: Three-, five-, or eight-pound dumbbells, depending on what feels comfortable to you.

Technique: With dumbbells, sit on the bench with your feet on the floor. Hold the dumbbells on top of your thighs. Your arms should be slightly

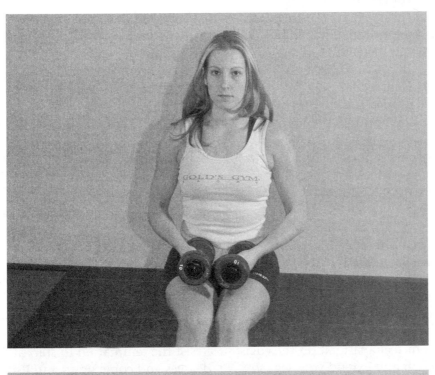

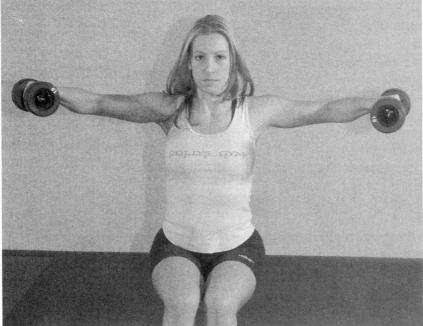

Dumbbell Lateral Raise

bowed. Lift the dumbbells up and out from your body in an arc until your arms are parallel to the floor. Make sure that your shoulders and shoulder blades remain stationary; they will pivot, but don't lift them up.

Sets and reps: Two sets of 10 to 12 repetitions.

Tip: To understand the correct motion for this exercise, imagine that your wrists are being pulled up by an invisible puppeteer.

Biceps Curl (illustrated on p. 66)

Follow the form described for this exercise in the beginner program, but add a little more weight. Remember to concentrate on form. Instead of two sets of 10 repetitions as before, do two sets of 12 to 15 repetitions.

Dips

Body area affected: Triceps.

Equipment needed: Two benches or two chairs.

Weight: Body weight.

Technique: Put two benches or chairs parallel to each other, about three or four feet apart. Sit on the edge of one bench and extend your legs so the heels of your feet rest on the other bench. Supporting your weight on your hands, gently slide your hips off the bench. Your knees should be slightly bent so that you are using your arms to support your weight. Slowly lower your body by bending your elbows. Keeping your body erect, push yourself back up by straightening your elbows. This exercise prepares you for Dips on parallel bars, which are more challenging because your legs are hanging free instead of resting on a bench.

Sets and reps: Initially, as many as you can do comfortably. This exercise may seem agonizing at first, so start with a low number of reps.

Tips: Keep your elbows as close to your torso as possible, and don't hyperextend your elbows when you

raise your body back up. Don't shorten the motion.

Pelvic Tilt and Crunches

Do these exercises in the same manner and order as you did them in the beginner program, but add one set of each exercise.

Balance Ball Crunch (illustrated on p. 78)

Body areas affected: Abdominals and trunk.

Equipment needed: Balance ball.

Weight: Body weight.

Technique: Start with the ball in the middle of your back, your body fully extended and parallel to the floor, both feet flat on the floor, and your hands and arms across your chest. Raise your upper body about 30 degrees, as you would for a normal crunch. Since this is a crunch, you don't do a full sit-up.

Sets and reps: Two sets of as many repetitions as you can comfortably do.

Tips: Stay fully extended at the start and raise your upper body 30 degrees. Resist the temptation to start at 30 degrees and come up to a full sit-up position.

Day 2: Legs, Chest, Shoulders, and Triceps

Wall Squats with Balance Ball (illustrated on p. 79)

Body areas affected: Quadriceps, hamstrings, and glutes.

Equipment needed: Balance ball.

Weight: Body weight.

Technique: Face away from the wall, with the ball between the wall and the small of your back. Your back should be flat, and your feet in front of you. Slowly squat down, making sure your upper body is perpendicular to the floor and not leaning. You should be able to squat lower than in a regular squat without a balance ball.

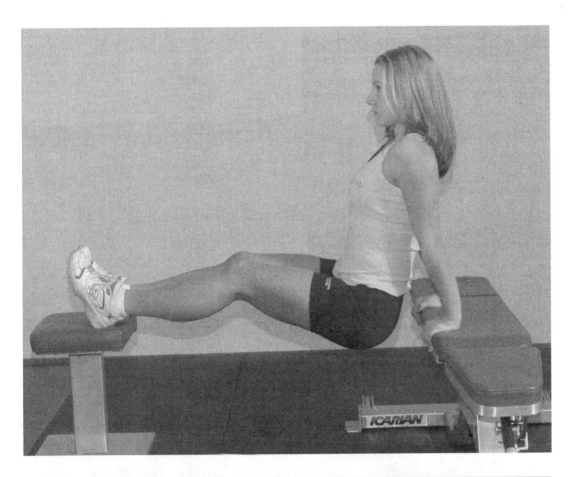

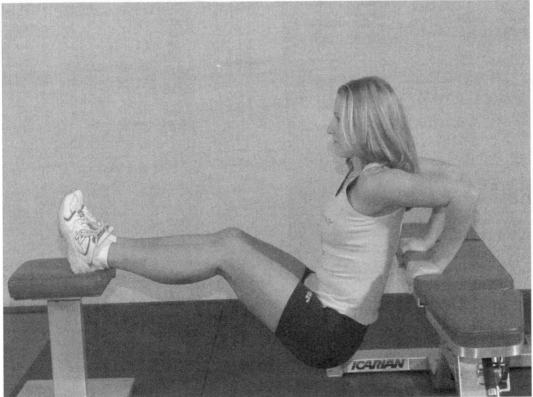

Dips

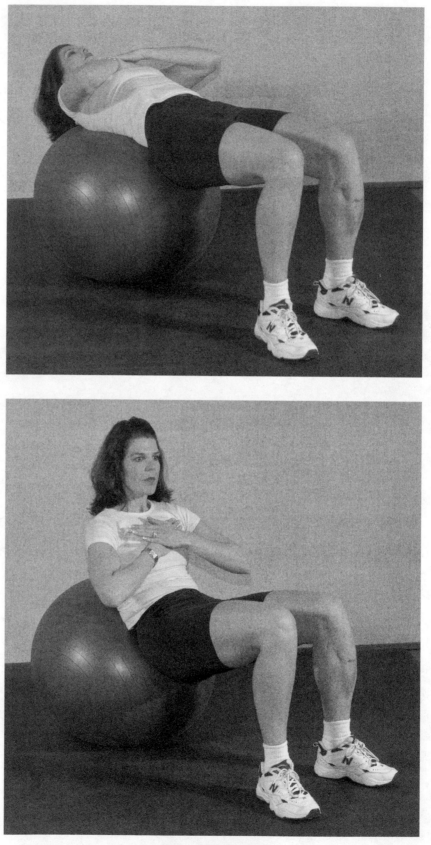

Balance Ball Crunch

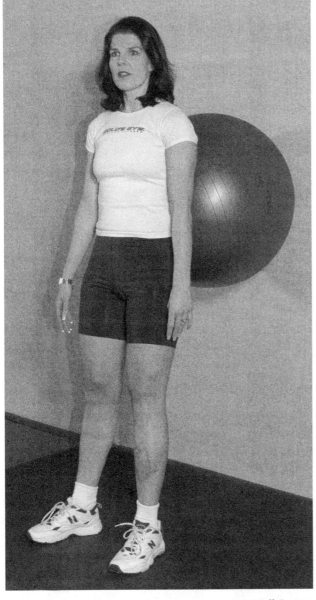 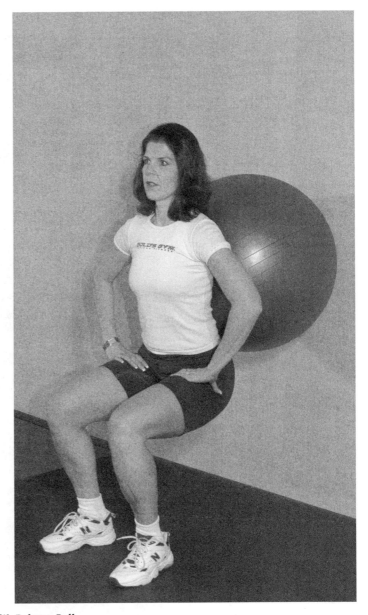

Wall Squats with Balance Ball

Sets and reps: Two sets of 12 repetitions; in the second set, add repetitions if you feel comfortable doing so.

Tip: Make sure that your knees do not extend over your toes; this would place too much stress on your knees.

Machine Bench Press (illustrated on p. 80)

Body areas affected: Pectoráls, deltoids, and triceps.

Equipment needed: Universal or Nautilus bench press machine.

Technique: Lie with your back flat on the bench and your feet flat on the floor. Grip the bars with your palms turned upward and your hands about shoulder-width apart. Using a fluid motion, lift the bar up and slightly back, so that the bar moves above your eyes as you extend your arms. Slowly lower the bar back to your chest.

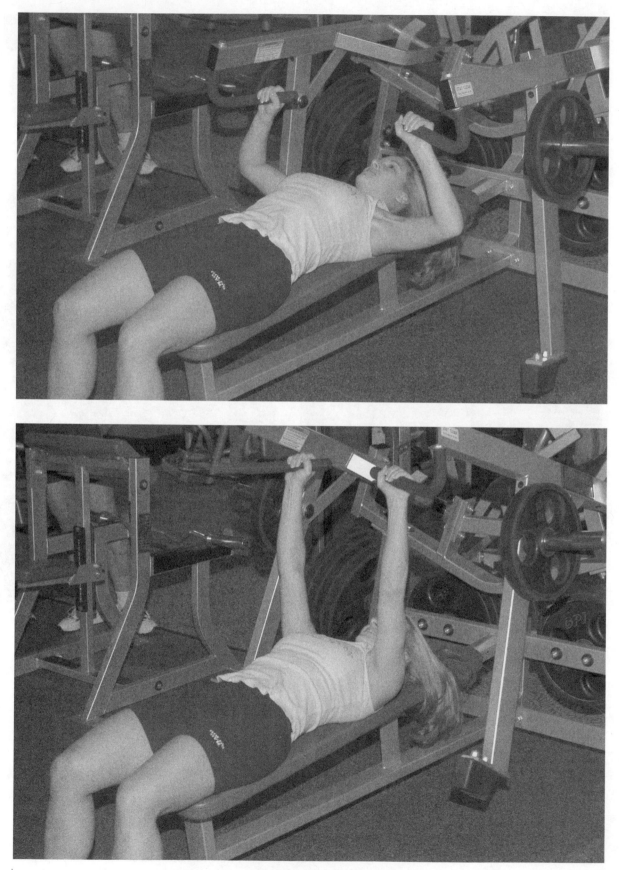

Machine Bench Press

Don't arch your back or neck while you are lifting, as this can cause injury.

Sets and reps: Two sets of 12 repetitions; in the second set, add repetitions if you feel comfortable doing so.

Tips: Start with the weight between your shoulders and chest. Try not to lock your elbows at the top of the motion.

Seated Calf

Body area affected: Calf muscles.

Equipment needed: Nautilus calf machine.

Technique: Sit with your back straight (not arched) and with your toes on the footpads. With the weights snug against your thighs, push upward with your toes so that your heels rise off the pads, then slowly lower your heels to the starting position.

Sets and reps: Two sets of 12 repetitions; in the second set, add repetitions if you feel comfortable doing so.

Hack Squats (on Machine)

(illustrated on p. 82)

Body areas affected: Quadriceps and glutes.

Equipment needed: Squat machine.

Technique: With your back flat against the machine, hold the weight

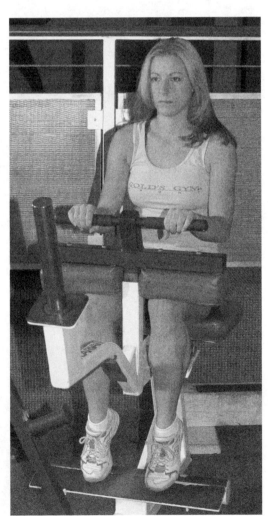

Seated Calf

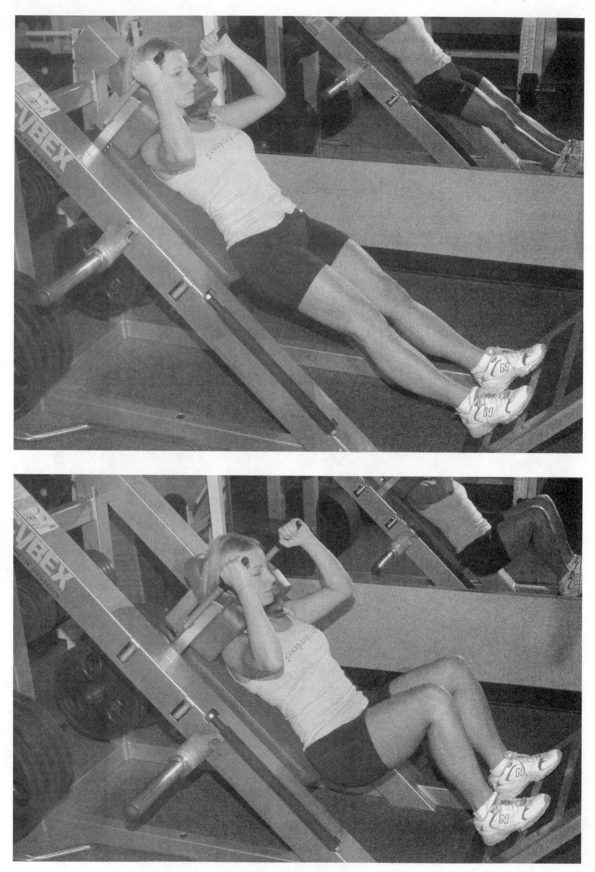

Hack Squats (on Machine)

with an overhand grip behind your body so that it is resting just below your buttocks. Slowly squat down until the weight is close to the floor, then straighten back up to the starting position.

Sets and reps: Weeks 1–2: Two sets of 12 repetitions. *Weeks 3–7:* Three sets of 12 repetitions; in the third set, add repetitions if you feel comfortable doing so.

Tips: Have your knees track your toes, that is, make sure that your toes are not splayed outward or turned inward. Keep your back as straight as possible (the machine will help you do this).

Preacher Curl

Body area affected: Biceps.

Equipment needed: Preacher bench and dumbbells or barbell, or preacher curl machine.

Technique: Rest your elbows and forearms on the preacher stand and fully extend your arms. Grasp the barbell or dumbbells with an underhand grip. Curl the weight as you would in the Biceps Curl until the bar almost touches your collarbone. Slowly return the barbell or dumbbells to the starting position.

Sets and reps: Weeks 1–2: Three sets of 10 repetitions. *Weeks 3–5:* Three sets of eight repetitions. *Weeks 6–7:* Three

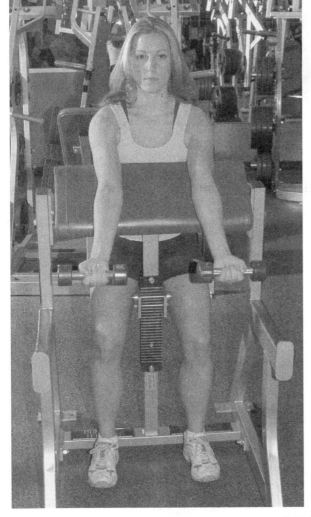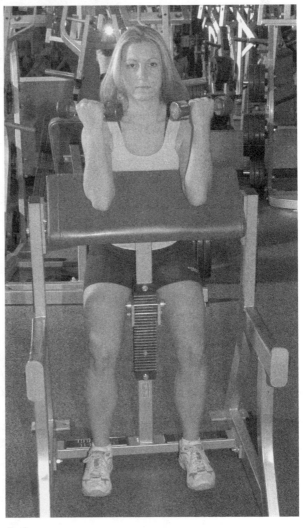

Preacher Curl

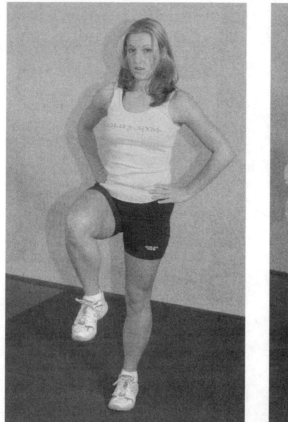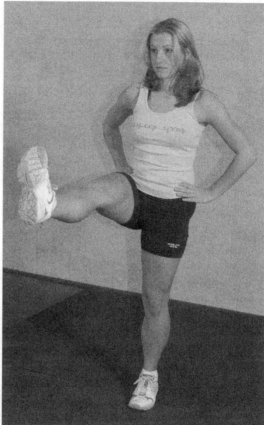

Balance Exercise . . .

sets of 12 repetitions; in the third set, add repetitions if you feel comfortable doing so.

Tip: Use light weight initially, since the design of the machine makes it difficult to cheat and use muscles other than your biceps.

Balance Exercise

Stand erect with your feet shoulder-width apart and your knees slightly bent. Slowly lift one leg off the floor, starting with the leg bent and then extending it straight forward. Hold your foot off the floor for a few seconds, then lower it to the starting position. Next, extend the leg to the side of your body, holding it for a few seconds. Next, extend one leg behind you off the floor. Repeat with your other leg.

Keep your leg two to three inches off the floor at the beginning of the exercise; gradually try to lift it higher as you become more comfortable with the exercise.

Cardiovascular Workout

Follow your workout with a cardio exercise. Exercise for at least 20 minutes at your target heart rate. Since you won't reach your target rate until at least five minutes into the exercise, consider adding five minutes or more to the length of your cardio workout in the beginner program. If you want to increase the intensity of the exercise (in speed or angle of incline, for instance), do so gradually.

Be sure to cool down and stretch after you finish your workout.

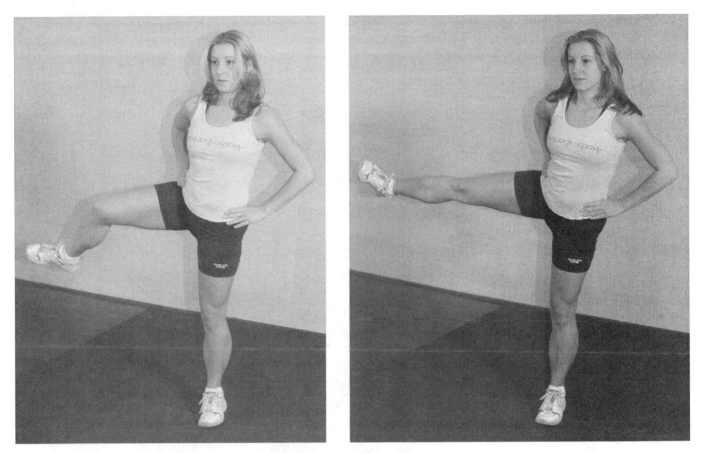

. . . Balance Exercise

Men's Beginner Workout

This six-week program features three workouts per week. Each day focuses on a different combination of body areas and muscle groups: The first day concentrates on your back, shoulders, and arms; the second day focuses on your legs, chest, shoulders, and triceps; and the third day focuses on your legs, back, chest, and biceps. In this way, you will work the same muscle group twice a week, but not three times, thus avoiding injury from overuse.

To determine how much weight you should use for each exercise, you need to determine your repetition maximum, or RM. This is simply the maximum weight that you can lift for a specific number of repetitions before exhaus-

tion. For instance, if the most you can bench-press 100 pounds is 10 times, then your 10-repetition maximum, or 10RM, is 100 pounds. You may be able to lift 120 pounds only six times, so your 6RM for the bench press is 120 pounds.

In the exercises that call for two sets of 12 reps, challenge yourself in the second set by trying to add a few more repetitions. If you can do four or more reps extra, increase the amount of weight for your next workout (but by no more than five percent at a time).

In the exercises that call for the maximum number of repetitions, do as many reps as you can do for the two sets of that exercise. You will develop an instinct for this the more you perform the exercises.

GOLD'S STARS

Paul, 47, systems engineer
Debby, 44, global salesperson

Going to the gym is a big part of the weekly schedule for Paul and Debby. Both of them work out several times a week, and they always find time in their busy schedules to include exercise.

Paul took up rowing 20 years ago and has been a dedicated fitness enthusiast ever since. He likes the feeling he gets in his muscles after a strenuous workout.

"Your muscles get a little tight, but it's a good feeling," he says. Paul also says that if he wasn't able to go to the gym, he'd find another physical activity to do.

Debby's story is about overcoming obstacles. Overweight as a child, she took up running in college and wound up becoming anorexic. She eventually started doing aerobics and was doing fine until a serious bicycle accident when she was in her 30s left her with a crushed left leg. For two years she underwent grueling physical therapy sessions four times a week and got back on her feet again. As if that were not enough adversity, she developed a degenerative disk condition in her back because one leg was shorter than the other as a result of the accident. That necessitated another eight months of physical therapy.

Today, she works out regularly, using an exercise program tailored specifically to her needs, and reaps the physical and emotional benefits, as well as the added benefit of keeping her various body parts in sync.

Happily, Debby's biggest problem seems to be reining herself in when she finds herself exercising too hard. "I always want to push it and do more than I should," she says. "I need to remember to limit myself."

Kim, 23, fitness consultant

As a former college cheerleader who now counsels people embarking on fitness programs, Kim knows that teamwork can be as important in the gym as it is on the basketball court or football field. That means, first of all, teaming up with a trainer to set up a specific program that will address your specific needs and goals. If going to the gym for the first time feels a little intimidating, that's normal, she says. But it's also easily overcome by working out with a friend or friends to help keep you motivated.

In her role as a fitness consultant, Kim interacts regularly with people who have never set foot in a gym before but have been told by their doctor that they need to develop a regular exercise program because their cholesterol level is too high, for instance, or because they need to lose weight. Then there are those who come in after the holidays when they notice they're starting to expand in the wrong direction.

"No one can really motivate you but you," Kim says, "except maybe your spouse. But when their pants don't fit, most people get the point."

Rest about 30 seconds to a minute between sets, and one to two minutes between exercises.

EXERCISES FOR WEEKS 1 AND 2
Day 1: Back, Shoulders, and Arms

Low Row

Body areas affected: Deltoids, upper back, trapezoids, and scapulas.

Equipment needed: Universal low row machine.

Technique: From a sitting position, with your arms extended, pull the weight toward your chest as you flex your elbows. Try not to lean forward. Keep your back straight, not arched. Slowly return the weight to the starting position.

Sets and reps: Two sets of 12 repetitions; in the second set, add repetitions if you feel comfortable doing so.

Tips: Keep your lower back straight. Pull with your elbows, not with your hands.

Lat Pull (illustrated on p. 88)

Body areas affected: Latissimus dorsi muscles (lats) and biceps.

Equipment needed: Lat machine.

Technique: Depending on the height of the machine and the length of the pulley, you can do this exercise while sitting on a padded chair or kneeling with your feet crossed behind you. Drop your head forward and keep your back straight. Raise your arms

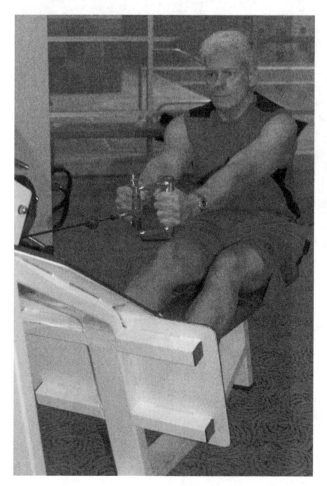
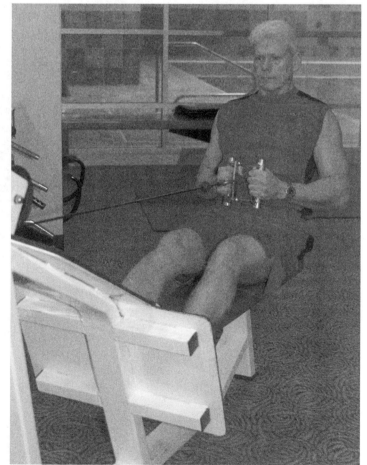

Low Row

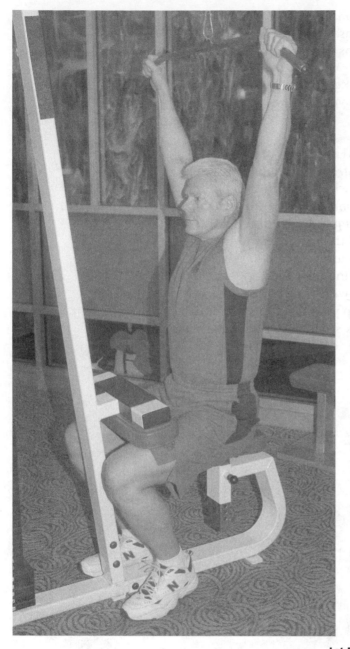 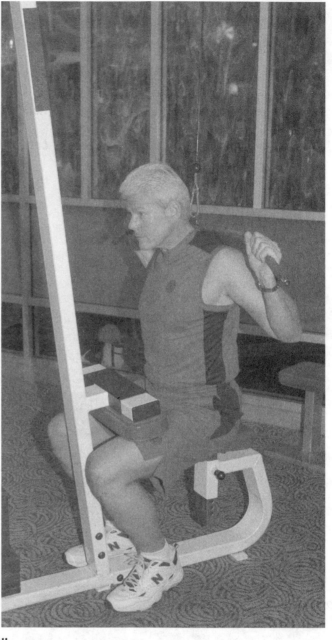

Lat Pull

and grab the bar above your head in an overhand grip; your hands should be about shoulder-width apart. Slowly pull the bar down toward the back of your neck, pulling your shoulder blades down first and then with your arms. To return to the starting position, slowly let the bar go back up—first with your arms, then with your shoulder blades.

Sets and reps: Two sets of 12 repetitions; in the second set, add repetitions if you feel comfortable doing so.

Tip: Concentrate on pulling down with your shoulder blades first, as this forces your lats to do the work. If you pull the weight down with your arms, the primary muscle used will be the biceps.

Balance Ball Crunch

Body areas affected: Abdominals and trunk.

Equipment needed: Balance ball.

Weight: Body weight.

Technique: Start with the ball in the middle of your back, your body fully extended and parallel to the floor, both feet flat on the floor, and your hands and arms across your chest. Raise your upper body about 30 degrees, as you would for a normal crunch. Since this is a crunch, you don't do a full sit-up.

Sets and reps: Two sets at the maximum number of reps you can comfortably do.

Tips: Stay fully extended at the start and raise your upper body 30 degrees. Resist the temptation to start at 30 degrees and come up to a full sit-up position.

Standing Row

Body areas affected: Deltoids, upper back, trapezoids, and scapulas.

Equipment needed: Dumbbells, barbell, or Universal machine with pulley attachment.

Technique: If you are using dumbbells, hold them in front of you with an overhand grip, keeping your hands close together. If you are using a barbell or bar attached to a pulley, hold it with an overhand grip, keeping your hands close enough together so that your thumbs would touch if you extended them. Standing erect with your knees slightly bent, exhale and pull the bar or dumbbells up near your body (parallel to your trunk) to about an inch below your chin. Hold for a second, then relax and slowly lower the bar or dumbbells.

Sets and reps: Two sets of 12 repetitions; in the second set, add repetitions if you feel comfortable doing so.

Tips: Keep your lower back straight, and make sure that your knees are slightly bent.

Triceps Pushdown (illustrated on p. 90)

Body area affected: Triceps.

Equipment needed: Lat machine or cable crossover machine.

Technique: Standing, grasp the bar with an overhand grip, with your hands close together, your elbows tight against your sides, and your forearms extended. Starting with the bar at about chest level, push it down, then slowly return it to the starting position.

Sets and reps: Two sets of 12 repetitions; in the second set, add repetitions if you feel comfortable doing so.

Tip: Keep your elbows as stationary as possible.

Biceps Curl

Body area affected: Biceps.

Equipment needed: Dumbbells, barbell, or biceps machine.

Technique: Stand erect with your feet shoulder-width apart. Hold the dumbbells with an underhand grip and let them rest against your thighs. Flex your right arm at the elbow, raise the dumbbell until it is a few inches from your chest, then lower it to the starting position. Repeat with your left arm. Go slowly, and continue to concentrate on your breathing.

Sets and reps: Two sets of 12 repetitions, alternating arms (12 right, 12 left, 12 right, 12 left). Alternating arms at each repetition wouldn't cause enough muscle fatigue in the arm. In the second set, add repetitions if you feel comfortable doing so.

Tips: The Biceps Curl looks easy to do but is often done incorrectly. To make sure that you are isolating your biceps, start the motion with your upper arms flush against your

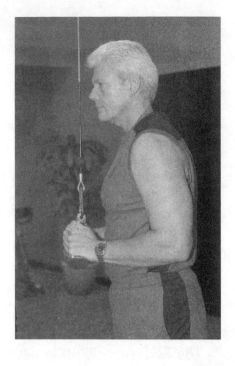 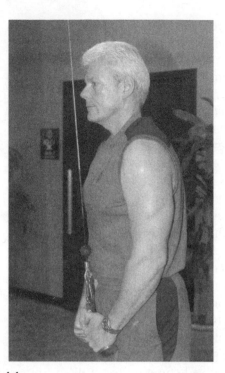

Triceps Pushdown

ribs. Keep your elbows and upper arm stationary through the entire motion.

Low Back Machine

Body area affected: Sacrospinalis muscle.

Equipment needed: Low back machine.

Technique: The machine is set up so you sit leaning forward with your upper back and lower back resting against separate pads and your feet on a small platform. There should be belts that you can fasten around your hips and legs. Starting in this position, push back with your upper back until your upper body is at about a 45-degree angle to the seat. Slowly return to the starting position.

Sets and reps: Two sets of 12 repetitions; in the second set, add repetitions if you feel comfortable doing so.

Tips: Don't arch your back at any time during the exercise. Don't hyperextend, or push too far back.

Day 2: Legs, Chest, Shoulders, and Triceps

Wall Squats with Balance Ball

Body areas affected: Quadriceps, hamstrings, and glutes.

Equipment needed: Balance ball.
Weight: Body weight.

Technique: Face away from the wall, with the ball between the wall and the small of your back. Your back should be flat, and your feet in front of you. Slowly squat down, making sure your upper body is perpendicular to the floor and not leaning. You should be able to squat lower than in a regular squat without a balance ball.

Sets and reps: Two sets of 12 repetitions; in the second set, add repetitions if you feel comfortable doing so.

Tip: Make sure that your knees do not extend over your toes; this would place too much stress on your knees.

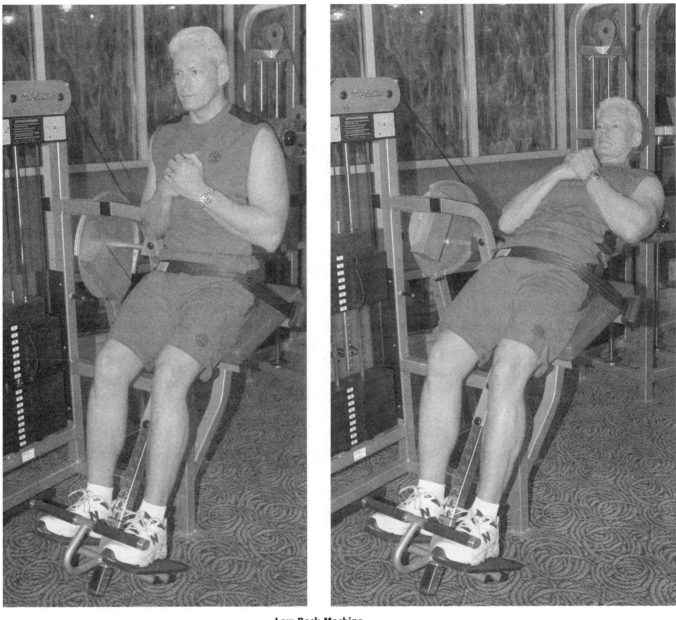

Low Back Machine

Machine Bench Press

Body areas affected: Pectorals, deltoids, and triceps.

Equipment needed: Universal or Nautilus bench press machine.

Technique: Lie with your back flat on the bench and your feet flat on the floor. Grip the bars with your palms turned upward and your hands about shoulder-width apart. Using a fluid motion, lift the bar up and slightly back, so that the bar moves above your eyes as you extend your arms. Slowly lower the bar back to your chest. Don't arch your back or neck while you are lifting, as this can cause injury.

Sets and reps: Two sets of 12 repetitions; in the second set, add repetitions if you feel comfortable doing so.

Tips: Start with the weight between your shoulders and chest. Don't lock your elbows at the top of the motion.

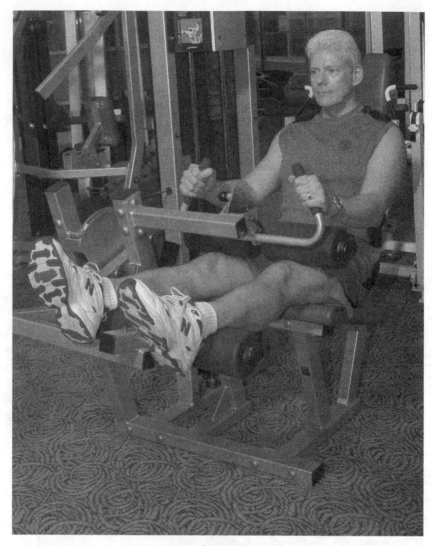

Seated Leg Curl...

Seated Leg Curl

Body area affected: Hamstrings.

Equipment needed: Nautilus leg curl machine.

Technique: Sit with your back flush against the padded back support and your calves on top of the leg pads. Use a seatbelt if one is available. Start with your legs extended and slowly flex them while holding on to the side bars. Hold and contract, then slowly bring your legs back up to the starting position.

Sets and reps: Two sets of 12 repetitions; in the second set, add repetitions if you feel comfortable doing so.

Tip: Don't arch your back.

Twisting Crunch

Body areas affected: Abdominals and obliques.

Equipment needed: Floor mat or any soft, flat surface.

Weight: Body weight.

Technique: Lie on your back on the floor with your hands crossed in front of your chest and your knees bent. Raise yourself up and twist so that you can touch your left knee with your

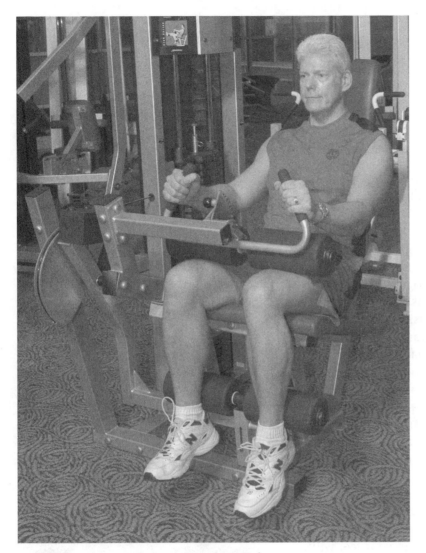

. . . Seated Leg Curl

right elbow. Lower yourself. Alternate with touching your right knee with your left elbow.

Sets and reps: Two sets of maximum repetitions.

Tips: Cross one foot over the opposite knee, so that only one knee will be bent. You can then raise the opposite elbow to touch that knee, and vice versa. If you have, or think you have, a lower back problem, don't do this exercise unless you are cleared by your physician or physical therapist. This caveat applies to any exercise that involves twisting.

Dumbbell Shoulder Raise
(illustrated on pp. 94–95)

Body area affected: Deltoids.

Equipment needed: Dumbbells.

Technique: Stand erect and hold the dumbbells against the top of your thighs at about pelvis height. Your arms should be slightly bowed. Lift the dumbbells up and out from your body in an arc until your upper arms are parallel to the floor. Make sure that your shoulders and shoulder blades remain stationary; they will pivot, but do not lift them up.

Sets and reps: Two sets of 12

repetitions; in the second set, add repetitions if you feel comfortable doing so.

Tip: To understand the correct motion for this exercise, imagine that your wrists are being pulled up by an invisible puppeteer.

Hanging Knee Raise

Body areas affected: Abdominals, hip flexors, and quadriceps.

Equipment needed: Pull-up bar or Universal hip flexor machine.

Weight: Body weight.

Technique: Hang from the pull-up bar with your legs together. Flex your knees and raise up as high as you can—to your chest, if possible, then extend your knees to the starting position. On the hip flexor machine, grip the handles and place your forearms on the pads. With your back against the padded back support, lift your knees up toward your chest, then extend them to the starting position.

Sets and reps: Two sets of maximum repetitions.

Tip: If you are using a pull-up bar, try to minimize the swinging of your body, as this will make the exercise more difficult. Crossing your feet will help minimize the swinging. You may have to stop between repetitions until you get the motion under control.

Seated Calf

Body area affected: Calf muscles.

Equipment needed: Nautilus calf machine.

Technique: Sit with your back straight (not arched) and with your toes on the footpads. With the weights snug against your thighs, push upward with your toes so that your heels rise off the pads, then slowly lower your heels to the starting position.

Sets and reps: Two sets of 12 repetitions; in the second set, add repetitions if you feel comfortable doing so.

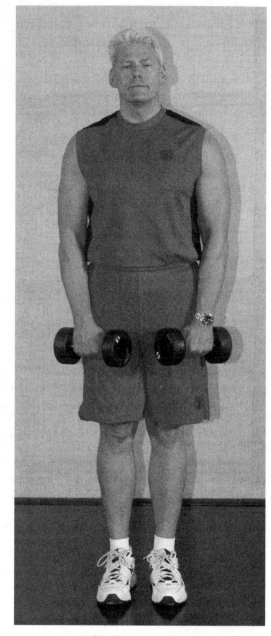

Dumbbell Shoulder Raise...

Pec Flye (illustrated on p. 96)

Body areas affected: Chest and biceps.

Equipment needed: Pec flye machine or dumbbells and bench.

Technique: If you're using a pec flye machine, sit with your back against the back support. Place your forearms behind the arm pads, with your upper arms parallel to the floor. Bring your arms together until the arm pads

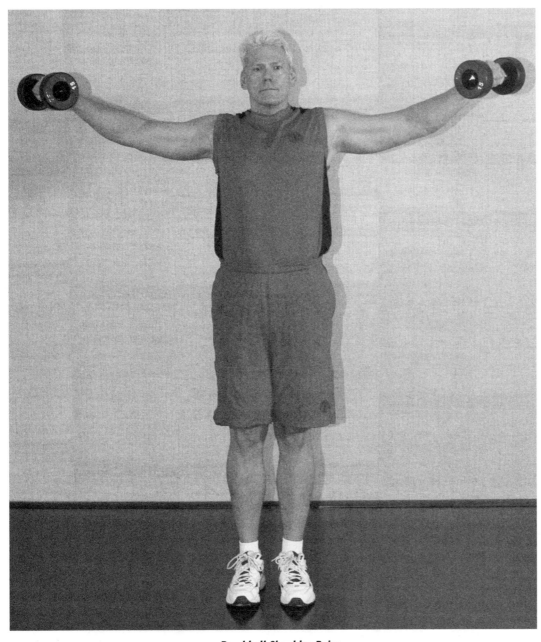

...Dumbbell Shoulder Raise

touch. Slowly return to the starting position. Throughout this exercise, force your lower back into the back support at all times, and don't arch your back.

If you're using dumbbells, lie with your back flat on the bench and your feet on the floor. Hold the dumbbells with an underhand grip at about chest level, with your arms extended parallel to the floor. Slowly bring the dumbbells together by raising your arms up and in, then slowly return to the starting position.

Throughout this exercise, force your lower back into the back support at all times, and try not to arch your back.

Sets and reps: Two sets of 12 repetitions; in the second set, add

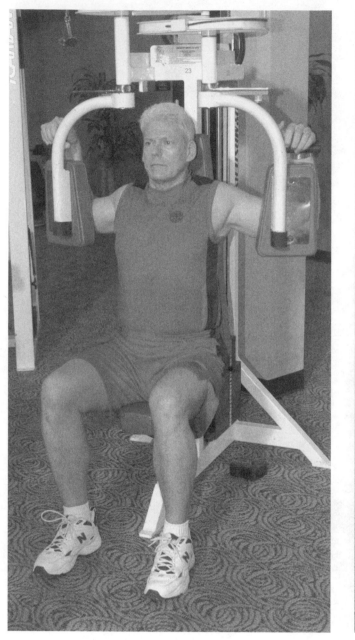 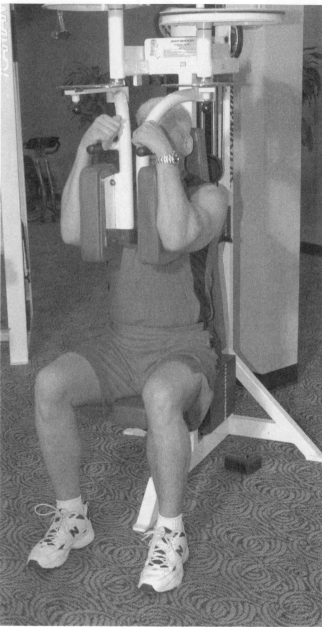

Pec Flye

repetitions if you feel comfortable doing so.

Tips: Flye machines vary in design, and you may use your hands or forearms to move the weight, depending on the model. Make sure that you are comfortable before you begin the exercise. Hold the contraction of each rep in this exercise.

Day 3: Legs, Back, Chest, and Biceps

Hip Abduction

Body area affected: Outer thigh muscles.

Equipment needed: Hip abductor/adductor machine. (You can also use ankle weights for this exercise.)

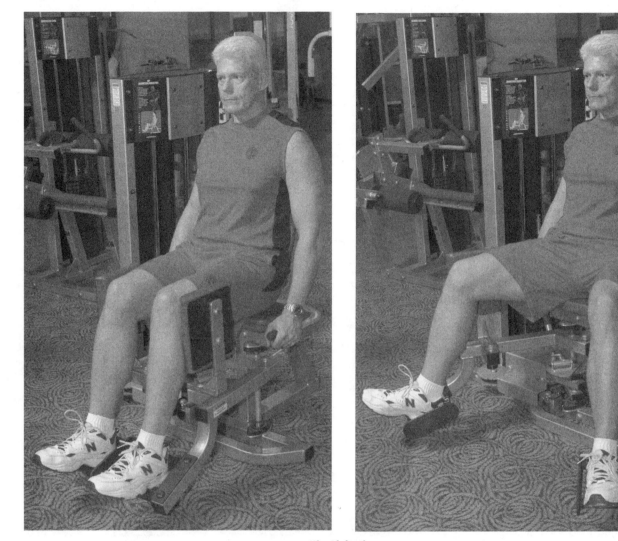

Hip Abduction

Technique: Sit with your upper and lower back flush against the back support of the machine. Use the seatbelt, if available, to keep your lower back from arching. Starting with your legs together, slowly push them outward, pause, and slowly bring them back together.

Sets and reps: Two sets of 12 repetitions; in the second set, add repetitions if you feel comfortable doing so.

Tips: Maintain good posture during this exercise, and don't arch your back. Keep your abdominal muscles tight. Try not to tense your neck muscles.

Hip Adduction (illustrated on p. 98)

Body area affected: Inner thigh muscles.

Equipment needed: Hip abductor/adductor machine. (You can also use ankle weights for this exercise.)

Technique: Sit with your upper and lower back flush against the back support of the machine. Use the seatbelt, if available, to keep your lower back from arching. Starting with your legs apart, slowly push them together, pause, and slowly spread them apart until they are in the starting position.

Sets and reps: Two sets of 12 repetitions; in the second set, add

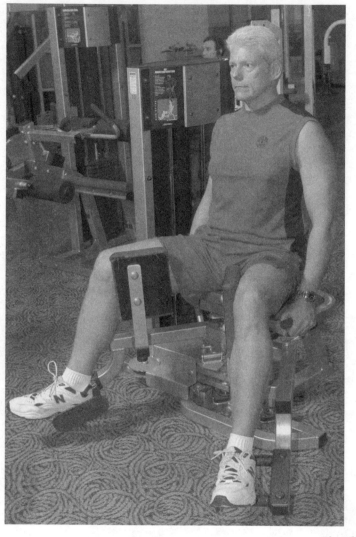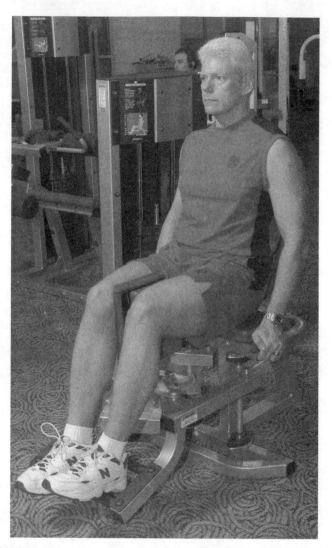

Hip Adduction

repetitions if you feel comfortable doing so.

Tips: Maintain good posture during this exercise, and don't arch your back. Keep your abdominal muscles tight. Try not to tense your neck muscles.

Weight-Assisted Pull-Ups

Body areas affected: Biceps, latissimus dorsi muscles (lats), and deltoids.

Equipment needed: Pull-up machine or Gravitron.

Technique: The machine allows you to do this exercise without having to lift your entire body weight. Adjust the weight on the machine to take some of the strain off your shoulders and arms. Kneel on the knee supports and grab the handles in a wide grip. Lean forward so that your head is in front of your arms and pull yourself up, then lower yourself down.

Sets and reps: Two sets of 12 repetitions; in the second set, add repetitions if you feel comfortable doing so.

Tip: The more weight you set the machine to, the easier it is to do the pull-up. Experiment to see which weight setting is right for you.

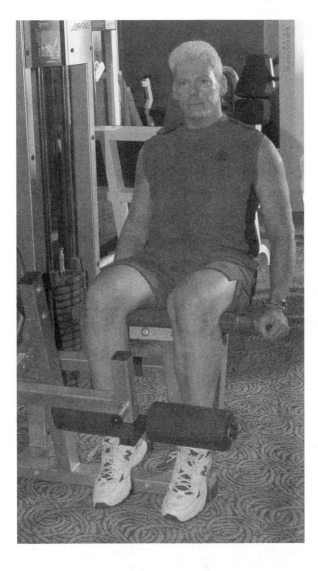
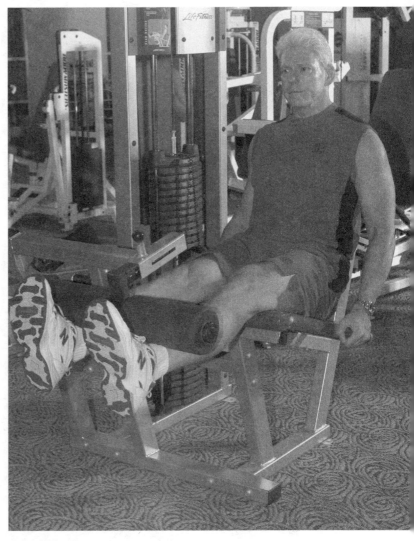

Leg Extension

Leg Extension

Body area affected: Quadriceps.

Equipment needed: Universal or Nautilus leg extension machine.

Technique: Keep your back flush against the seat; use a seatbelt if one is available. Your knees should be off the edge of the seat. Lift the weight by extending your knees until they are fully extended at the top of the motion. Contract the muscle and hold for two seconds, then slowly return to the starting position.

Sets and reps: Two sets of 12 repetitions; in the second set, add repetitions if you feel comfortable doing so.

Tip: On the return motion, be sure to keep your feet in a flexed position with your toes up. If your toes are pointed, you will put undue pressure on your patellar tendon (the tendon in front of and below your kneecap).

Knee Raise (on Apparatus)
(illustrated on p. 100)

Body areas affected: Abdominals, hip flexors, and quadriceps.

Equipment needed: Hip flexor apparatus or parallel bars.

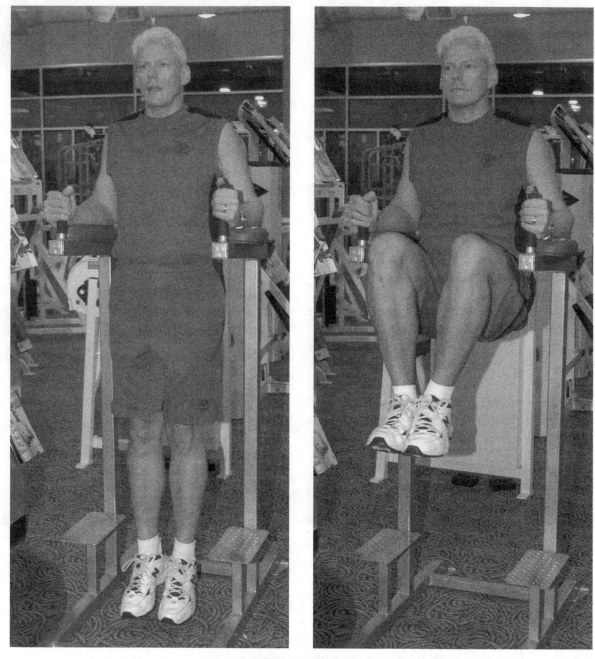

Knee Raise (on Apparatus)

Weight: Body weight.

Technique: Standing, grab the handles and place your forearms on the pads. With your back against the padded support, lift and flex your knees up toward your chest, then lower your knees until they are just below the level of your hips.

Sets and reps: Two sets of maximum repetitions.

Tip: To add difficulty to this exercise, perform the raise with your lower body in a pike position—with your legs fully extended and at a 90-degree angle to your body (to form an L shape).

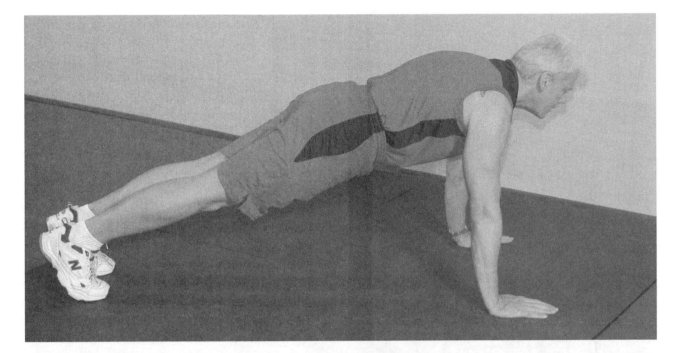

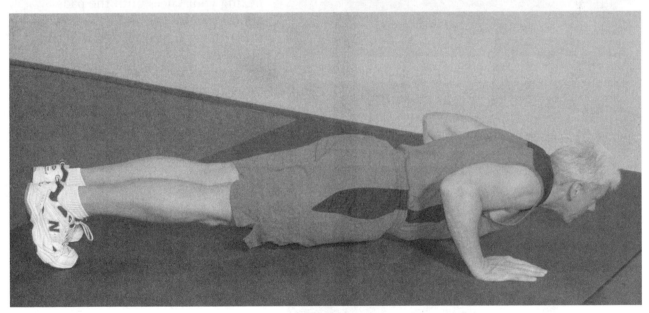

Push-Ups

Push-Ups

Body areas affected: Pectorals, biceps, and triceps.

Equipment needed: Floor mat or flat, nonslippery surface.

Weight: Body weight.

Technique: Get into the standard push-up position, raised up on your arms with your legs extended and your feet together. Try not to lock your arms in this position. Slowly lower yourself until your nose is nearly touching the floor, then raise yourself back up by pushing with your arms. Keep your back flat throughout the exercise.

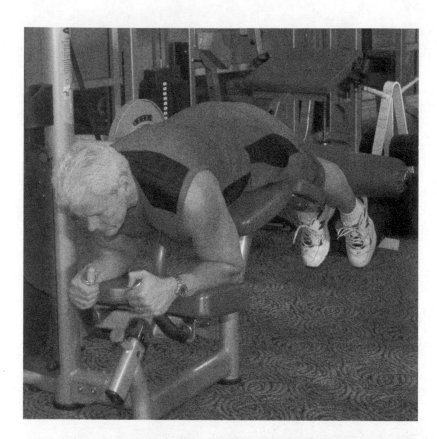

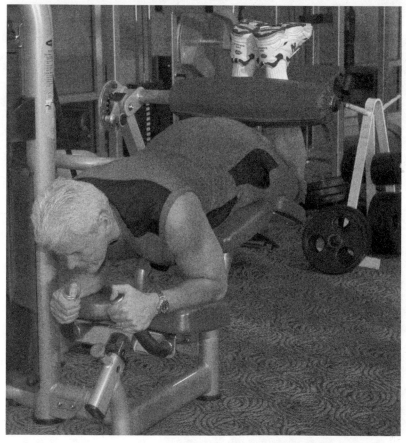

Leg Curl

Sets and reps: Two sets of maximum repetitions.

Tips: Go slowly—this will help you get the full benefit of the exercise. Changing the position of your hands—by positioning them farther apart or closer together, for example—will isolate a different part of your pectoral muscles.

Leg Curl

Body area affected: Hamstrings.

Equipment needed: Leg curl machine.

Technique: Lie face down on the bench with your kneecaps off the end and the backs of your lower legs touching the pads. With your hands holding the bars, lift the weight by flexing your knees until the pads almost touch your buttocks. Slowly lower the weight back to the starting position.

Sets and reps: Two sets of 12 repetitions; in the second set, add repetitions if you feel comfortable doing so.

Tips: Don't arch your back. Lie flat on the bench as much as possible.

Back Extension

Body areas affected: Lower back and abdominal muscles.

Equipment needed: Weight plate and bench or Universal, Nautilus, or similar machine.

Technique: Sit on a bench and hold a weight plate against your chest. Lean forward as far as you can, then raise yourself back up. On a Universal machine, lie face down on the back extension bench so that your upper body extends over the edge. Place your hands behind your neck (or hold a weight plate against your chest) and slowly lower your torso as far as you can. Slowly lift your torso back up until it is in line with your lower body. On a Nautilus machine, sit on the padded seat with your chest against the padded roller that provides resistance. With

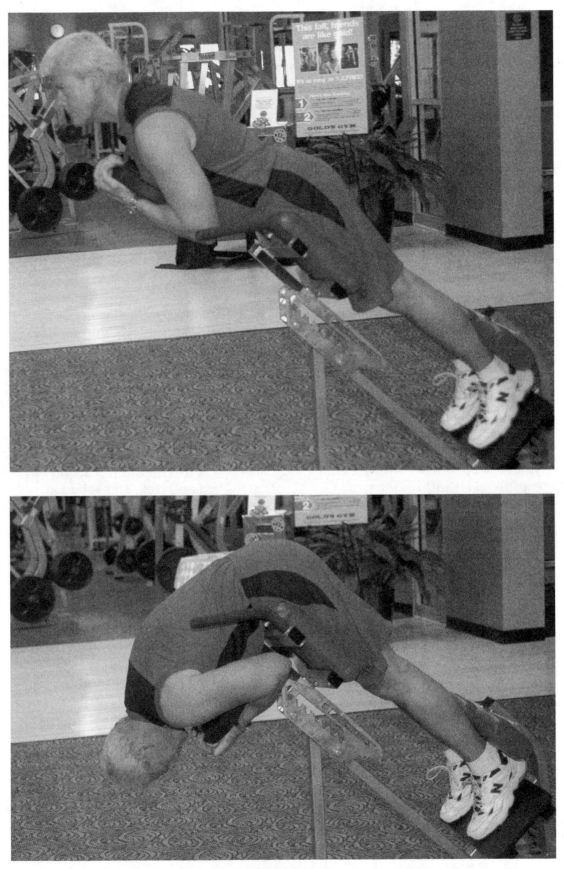

Back Extension

your hands crossed in front of you, move the weight forward by pressing with your chest.

Sets and reps: Two sets of 12 repetitions; in the second set, add repetitions if you feel comfortable doing so.

Tips: If you are new to this exercise, it is probably better to use a machine instead of the weight plate. If you have a lower back problem, don't do this exercise unless you are cleared by your physician or physical therapist.

Seated Twist with Medicine Ball

Body areas affected: Abdominal muscles and obliques.

Equipment needed: Medicine ball, plus workout mat or flat, nonslippery surface.

Technique: Sit on the floor in a crunch position with your knees bent and your feet on the floor. Holding the medicine ball with both hands, twist to either side and touch the ball to the floor. To add difficulty after you have become accustomed to this exercise, do it with your feet slightly off the floor.

Sets and reps: Two sets of maximum repetitions.

Tip: A twisting exercise may be harmful to your back if you already have a back problem or injury. If you have such an problem or injury, don't do this exercise unless you are cleared by your physician or physical therapist.

EXERCISES FOR WEEKS 3 THROUGH 6

After you have completed the first two weeks of the beginner program, perform three sets of all exercises, and add repetitions to the third set if you feel comfortable doing so. For the body weight exercises that call for two sets of maximum repetitions in weeks 1 and 2, perform three sets in weeks 3 through 6. Maintain the same rest period between sets and exercises.

MEN'S INTERMEDIATE WORKOUT

The intermediate workout follows the same logical pattern as the beginner workout, focusing on specific body parts for two of the three days. For example, you will do back exercises on the first and third days, shoulder exercises on the first and second days, and leg exercises on the second and third days. The intermediate program is seven weeks long, compared to six weeks for the beginner program.

Pay particular attention to the number of sets and repetitions, as they vary from exercise to exercise and from week to week. For example, on Day 2 of the first two weeks you will do two sets of 12 Leg Curl repetitions, on Day 2 of Weeks 3 and 4 you will do two sets of 10, and for Weeks 5 through 7 the number of repetitions drops to eight. One reason for this decrease is that at the same time your Leg Curl repetitions are decreasing, you are doing more Step-ups—sets of 12 the first two weeks, then 15, then 17, until you are doing 20 in the final week. This variation proves the value of a workout log.

As in the beginner workout, for the exercises where you will be doing three sets of a prescribed number of repetitions, add repetitions in the third set if you feel comfortable doing so. If you can do four or more additional repetitions, increase the amount of weight for your next workout (but by no more than five percent).

The amount of weight you use for each exercise should be based on your repetition maximum, or RM, for that exercise. (For instructions on how to determine your RM for a particular exercise, see page 85.)

For intermediate workouts, allow a longer rest period between sets than you did in the beginner workout— between one and two minutes. Allow one to two minutes of rest between exercises.

Day 1: Back, Shoulders, and Arms

Single Row with Dumbbell
(illustrated on pp. 106–107)

Body areas affected: Shoulders, upper back, and biceps.

Equipment needed: Dumbbell and bench.

Technique: Stand with one knee on the bench and the opposite foot on the floor. While gripping the end of the bench, hold the dumbbell in your free hand, making sure to keep your back straight and your shoulders square. Start with your arm extended and lift the dumbbell up as high as you can while bending your elbow, then lower it back down. Repeat with your other arm.

Sets and reps: Weeks 1–2: Three sets of 12 repetitions. *Weeks 3–4:* Three sets of 10 repetitions. *Weeks 5–7:* Three sets of 8 repetitions. In the third set, add repetitions if you feel comfortable doing so.

Tip: If you have a lower back problem, consult with a trainer or physical therapist before attempting this exercise.

Crunches

Body areas affected: Trunk and abdominal muscles.

Equipment needed: Workout mat or flat, nonslippery surface.

Weight: Body weight.

Technique: Lie on your back with your knees bent and your feet flat on the floor. Clasp your hands across your chest and slowly curl your trunk upward by raising your chest and shoulders off the floor. Keep your lower back firmly on the floor.

Sets and reps: Weeks 1–2: Three sets of 12 repetitions. *Week 3:* Three sets of 25 repetitions. *Weeks 4–5:* Three sets of 30 repetitions. *Weeks 6–7:* Three sets of 35 repetitions. In the third set, add repetitions if you feel comfortable doing so.

Tips: Go slowly. Take four seconds to lift up and four seconds to lower yourself back down. To add difficulty once you have mastered the exercise, hold a weight plate on your chest as you raise and lower yourself.

Shoulder Press with Dumbbells

Body area affected: Deltoids.

Equipment needed: Dumbbells and (optional) bench.

Technique: This exercise can be done from a standing or sitting position. Use a bench with a backrest if you are sitting; if there is no backrest, be sure to maintain good posture. Hold the dumbbells with an overhand grip with your palms turned forward. Start with your elbows flexed and the dumbbells level with your ears. Slowly raise the dumbbells and bring them together above your head, pause, then lower them back to the starting position.

Sets and reps: Weeks 1–2: Three sets of 12 repetitions. *Weeks 3–4:* Three sets of 10 repetitions. *Weeks 5–7:* Three sets of 8 repetitions. In the third set, add repetitions if you feel comfortable doing so.

Tips: It is risky if the dumbbells go below the level of your ears. Don't fully extend your elbows when you reach the top of the motion, and don't touch the dumbbells together. Keep your back straight, not arched.

Reverse Crunch (illustrated on p. 108)

Body area affected: Abdominal muscles.

Equipment needed: Workout mat or flat, nonslippery surface.

Weight: Body weight.

Technique: Lie on your back with your hands and your head forming a triangle (arms spread away from your sides). Lift your legs straight up off the floor and extend them so that your body forms an L shape. Keep your upper back and head against the

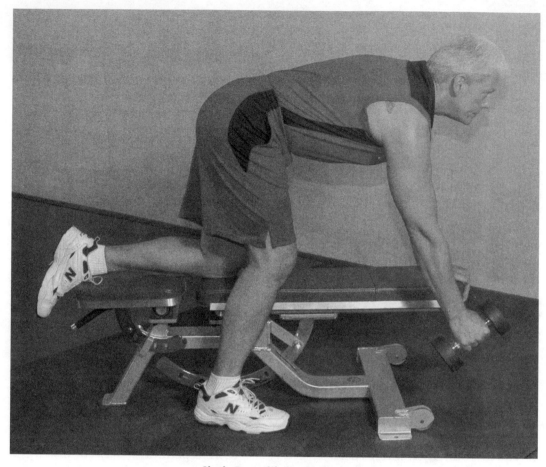

Single Row with Dumbbell . . .

floor. Using your lower abdominals, push up to get your buttocks off the floor and lift your legs higher.

Sets and reps: *Weeks 1–2:* Two sets of 12 repetitions. *Weeks 3–7:* Three sets of 15 repetitions. In the third set in Weeks 3 through 7, add repetitions if you feel comfortable doing so.

Tips: This is a difficult exercise to master. The most important thing to remember is to not arch your lower back. Imagine that you have a string tied to your pelvis, with the other end held above you. As the string is pulled from above, you move your pelvis straight up. In the first part of the exercise, your tailbone should not come off the floor.

Biceps Curl

Body area affected: Upper arms.

Equipment needed: Dumbbells.

Technique: Stand erect with your feet shoulder-width apart. Hold the dumbbells with an underhand grip and let them rest against your thighs. Flex your right arm at the elbow, raise the dumbbell until it is a few inches from your chest, then lower it to the starting position. Repeat with your left arm. Go slowly, and continue to concentrate on your breathing.

Sets and reps: *Weeks 1–2:* Three sets of 12 repetitions (12 right, 12 left, 12 right, 12 left—alternating arms at each repetition wouldn't cause enough muscle fatigue in the arm). *Weeks 3–4:* Three sets of 10 repetitions. *Weeks 5–7:*

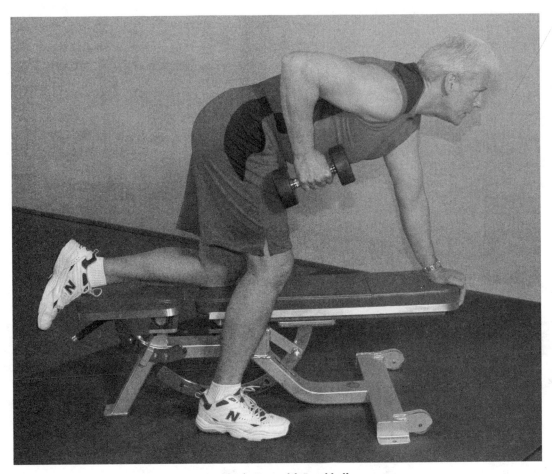

...Single Row with Dumbbell

Three sets of 8 repetitions. In the third set, add repetitions if you feel comfortable doing so.

Tip: The Biceps Curl looks easy to do but is often done incorrectly. To make sure that you are isolating your biceps, start the motion with your upper arms flush against your ribs. Keep your elbows and upper arm stationary all the way through the motion.

Triceps Extension (illustrated on p. 109)
   Body area affected: Triceps.
   Equipment needed: Bench and EZ curl bar or barbell, or pulley machine.
   Technique: You can sit on a padded chair (in which case the exercise is also called French Curls) or use a bench. When seated, hold the barbell with a close grip and bring the bar from behind your head to a position directly over your head, then return to the starting position.

On a bench, start with the bar just above your forehead and raise the bar, straightening your arms until they are extended so that the weight is above your chest. When using a pulley machine, grasp the bar with an over-hand grip and with your elbows bent at 90 degrees and tucked against body. Push down until your arms are extended.

Sets and reps: Weeks 1–2: Three sets of 12 repetitions. *Weeks 3–4:* Three sets of 10 repetitions. *Weeks 5–7:*

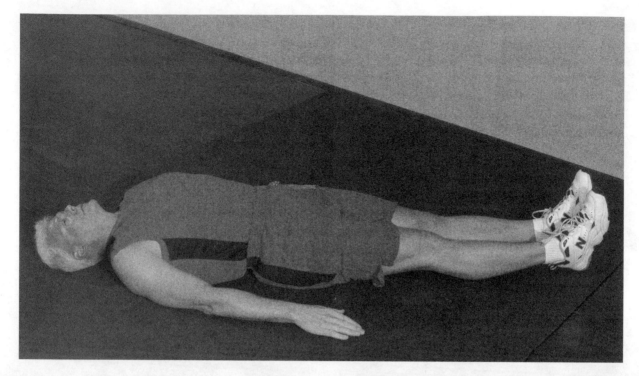

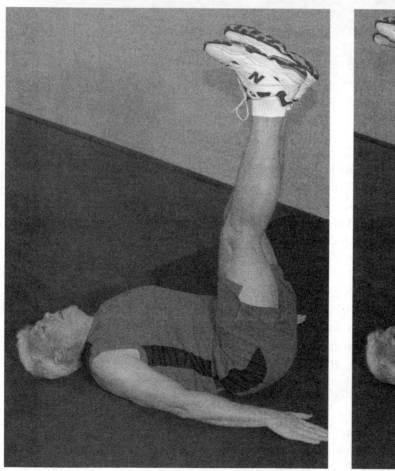

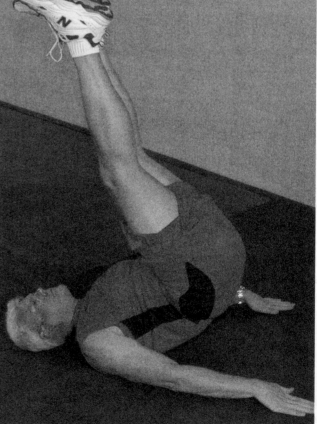

Reverse Crunch

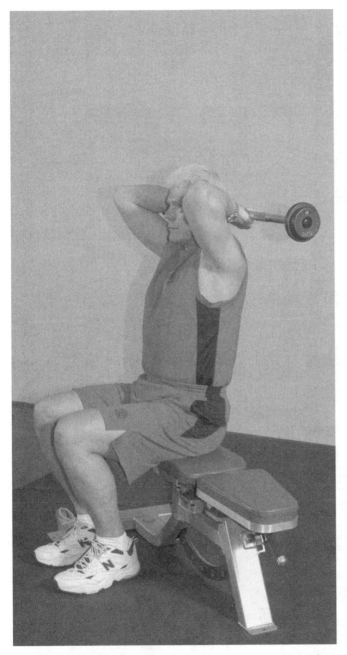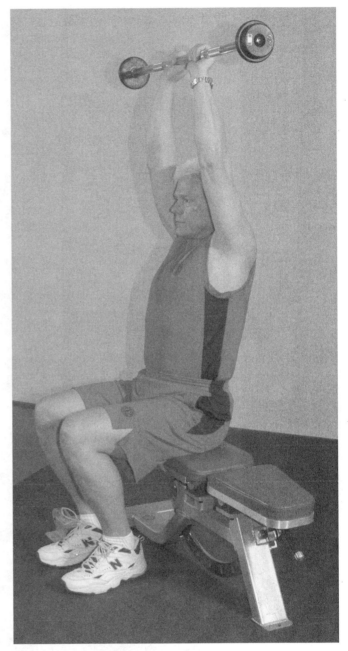

Triceps Extension

Three sets of 8 repetitions. In the third set, add repetitions if you feel comfortable doing so.

Tip: Be especially careful not to use too much weight in this exercise; if you lose control of the weight when it is above your head, neck, or chest, you could seriously injure yourself.

Day 2: Legs, Shoulders, and Triceps

Leg Press (illustrated on p. 110)
   Body areas affected: Lower legs and glutes.
   Equipment needed: Universal or Nautilus leg press machine.
   Technique: Sit in the chair and place your feet on the footpads. Keep your

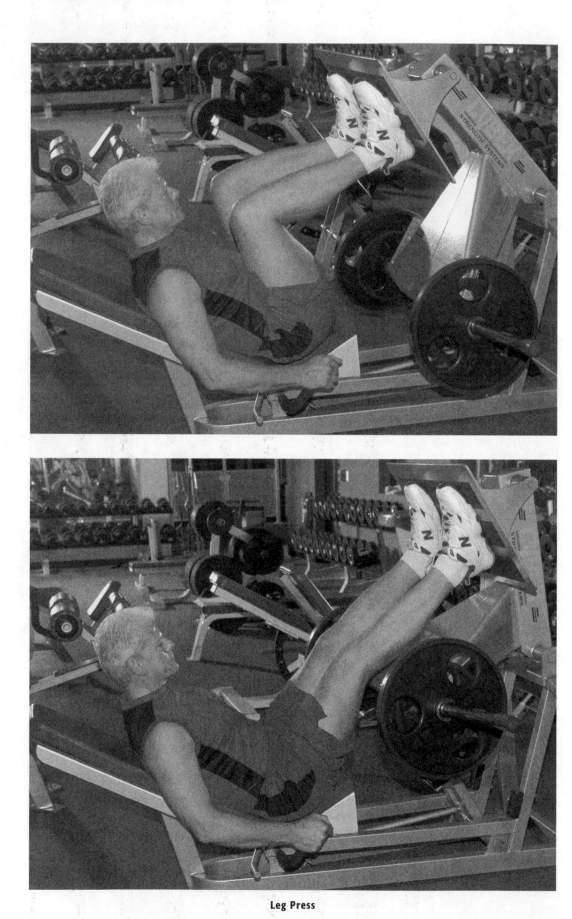

Leg Press

hips flat against the seat, and focus on going slowly. Push against the weight until your legs are almost fully extended. Slowly return to the starting position by bending your knees.

Sets and reps: *Weeks 1–2:* Three sets of 12 repetitions. *Weeks 3–4:* Three sets of 10 repetitions. *Weeks 5–7:* Three sets of 8 repetitions. In the third set, add repetitions if you feel comfortable doing so.

Tips: Have a trainer set up the chair correctly for your height and body type. When you do the eccentric (second) half of the motion, your feet should not be behind your knees, or you will place too much stress on your knees. Don't lock your knees at the top of the motion. Make sure that your knees track your toes, that is, that your feet are not splayed outward or pointed inward.

Bench Press (illustrated on p. 112)

Body areas affected: Pectorals, biceps, deltoids, and triceps.

Equipment needed: Bench and barbell.

Technique: Lie with your back flat on the bench and your feet flat on the floor. Rest the bar lightly on your chest and grasp it with your palms turned upward and your hands about shoulder-width apart. Using a fluid motion, lift the bar up and slightly back, so that the bar is above your eyes when your arms are at full extension. Slowly lower the bar back to your chest.

Sets and reps: *Weeks 1–2:* Two sets of 12 repetitions. *Weeks 3–7:* Three sets of 12 repetitions. In the third set, add repetitions if you feel comfortable doing so.

Tip: To avoid injury, don't arch your back or neck while you are lifting.

Twisting Sit-Ups

Body areas affected: Abdominal muscles and obliques.

Equipment needed: Exercise mat or flat, nonslippery surface.

Weight: Body weight.

Technique: Lie on your back with your hands crossed in front of your chest, your knees bent, and your feet flat on the floor. Raise yourself up and twist so that you touch your left knee with your right elbow. Lower yourself. Alternate with touching your right knee with your left elbow.

Sets and reps: Three sets of maximum repetitions.

Tip: Sit-ups may be harder on your lower back than crunches, and any twisting motion will have the same effect. Be extremely careful when doing this exercise if you have a lower back problem, and consult with your physician or physical therapist—who may tell you not to do it at all.

Leg Curl (illustrated on p. 102)

Body area affected: Hamstrings.

Equipment needed: Leg curl machine.

Technique: Lie face down on the bench with your kneecaps off the end and the backs of your lower legs touching the pads. With your hands holding the bars, lift the weight by flexing your knees until the pads almost touch your buttocks. Slowly lower the weight back to the starting position.

Sets and reps: *Weeks 1–2:* Two sets of 12 repetitions. *Weeks 3–4:* Two sets of 10 repetitions. *Weeks 5–7:* Two sets of 8 repetitions. In the second set, add repetitions if you feel comfortable doing so.

Tips: Don't arch your back. Lie flat on the bench as much as possible.

Dumbbell Shoulder Shrugs

Body areas affected: Trapezius, rhomboids, and deltoids.

Equipment needed: Dumbbells.

Technique: Start with the dumbbells at your sides, holding them in an over-

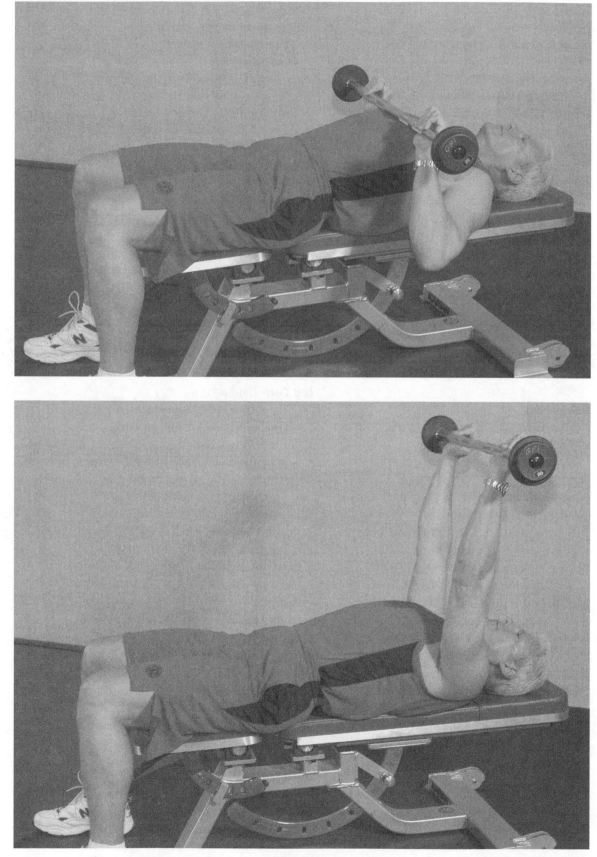

Bench Press

hand grip. Stand erect, with your knees slightly bent. Lift your shoulders toward your head—as if you are shrugging—and rotate them back slightly before returning to the starting position.

This exercise can also be done on a Universal bench press machine; face the bar and use the same motion.

Sets and reps: Weeks 1–2: Two sets of 12 repetitions. *Week 3:* Two sets of 10 repetitions. *Weeks 4–5:* Three sets of 12 repetitions. *Weeks 6–7:* Three sets of 10 repetitions. In the third set, add repetitions if you feel comfortable doing so.

Tips: This exercise is easy to do incorrectly, because it is tempting to use your wrists or arms to raise the weight. Concentrate on isolating your shoulders and making them do the work. Don't bend your elbows.

Step-Ups (illustrated on p. 114)

Body areas affected: Quadriceps, hamstrings, glutes, arms, and shoulders.

Equipment needed: Step-up box (one to two feet high) and dumbbells.

Technique: From a standing position, lean forward and step up on the box with one leg, then bring your other leg up onto the box. Step back down. Once you have mastered this motion and feel comfortable, hold dumbbells at your sides while you do the exercise.

Sets and reps: Weeks 1–2: Two sets of 12 repetitions. *Weeks 3–4:* Two sets of 15 repetitions. *Weeks 5–6:* Two sets of 17 repetitions. *Week 7:* Two sets of 20 repetitions.

Tip: Go slowly when you are learning this exercise. Balance is critical; you must get used to supporting yourself on one leg that is higher than the floor.

Seated Twist with Medicine Ball

Body areas affected: Abdominal muscles and obliques.

Equipment needed: Medicine ball, plus workout mat or flat, nonslippery surface.

Technique: Sit on the floor in a crunch position with your knees bent and your feet on the floor. Holding the medicine ball with both hands, twist to either side and touch the ball to the floor. To add difficulty after you have become accustomed to this exercise, do it with your feet slightly off the floor.

Sets and reps: Two sets of maximum repetitions.

Tip: A twisting exercise may be harmful to your back if you already have a back problem or injury. If you have such an problem or injury, don't do this exercise unless you are cleared by your physician or physical therapist.

Triceps Kickback (illustrated on p. 115)

Body area affected: Triceps.

Equipment needed: Bench and dumbbells.

Technique: Stand with one knee on the bench and the opposite foot on the floor. While gripping the end of the bench and holding the dumbbell in your free hand close to your side, bend over from the waist with your elbow held high so that your upper arm is parallel to the floor. Starting with your elbow at a 90-degree angle, fully extend your arm behind you. Slowly return to the starting position. Repeat with your other arm.

Sets and reps: Weeks 1–2: Three sets of 12 repetitions. *Weeks 3–4:* Three sets of 10 repetitions. *Weeks 5–7:* Three sets of 8 repetitions. In the third set, add repetitions if you feel comfortable doing so.

Tips: Imagine that you are a relay runner receiving a baton, and you will have a mental image of this exercise. Keep your back straight, and don't move the rest of your body as you do this exercise—move only your arm. Keep your eyes fixed downward; raising your head can strain your neck muscles.

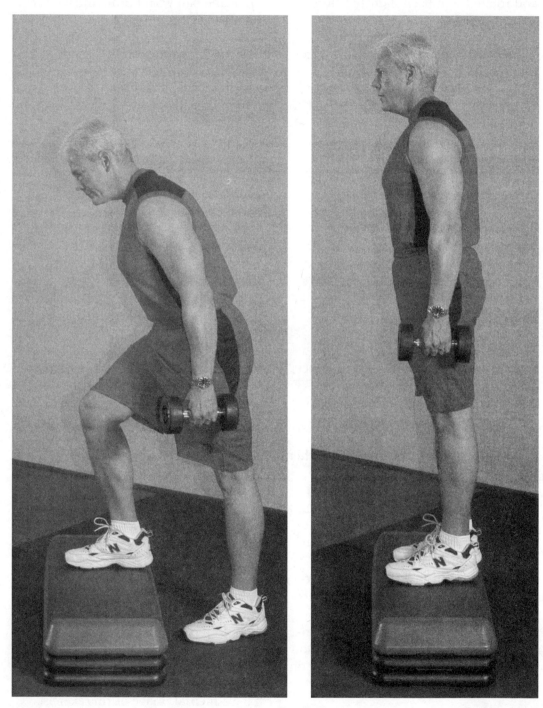

Step-Ups

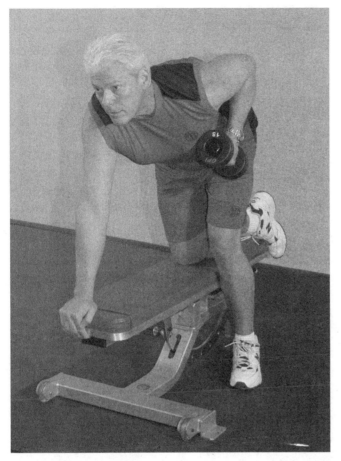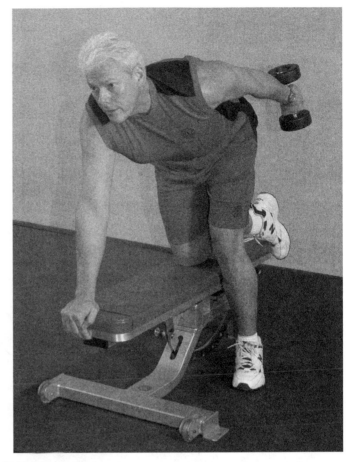

Triceps Kickback

Day 3: Legs, Back, Chest, and Biceps

Hack Squats (on Machine)

Body areas affected: Quadriceps and glutes.

Equipment needed: Squat machine.

Technique: With your back flat against the machine, hold the weight with an overhand grip behind your body so that it is resting just below your buttocks. Slowly squat until the weight is close to the floor, then straighten back up to the starting position.

Sets and reps: Weeks 1–2: Two sets of 12 repetitions. *Weeks 3–7:* Three sets of 12 repetitions. In the third set, add repetitions if you feel comfortable doing so.

Tips: Have your knees track your toes, that is, make sure that your toes are not splayed outward or turned inward. Keep your back as straight as possible (the machine will help you do this).

Pull-Ups (illustrated on p. 116)

Body areas affected: Biceps and latissimus dorsi muscles (lats).

Equipment needed: Pull-up bar.

Weight: Body weight.

Technique: Grab the bar with your palms turned forward and let your body hang from the bar. Lift yourself up so that your chin is above the level of the bar. If you have difficulty, place a box under the bar that is high enough for you to reach the bar comfortably. This exercise may also

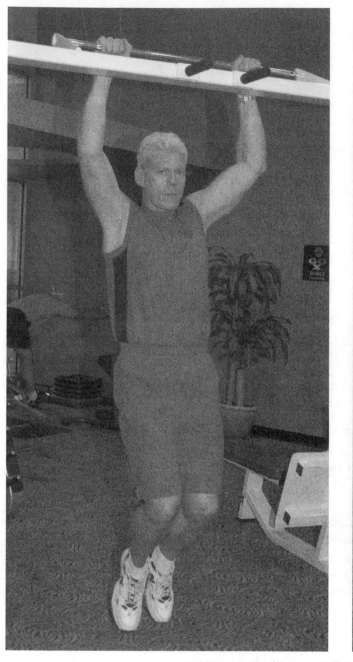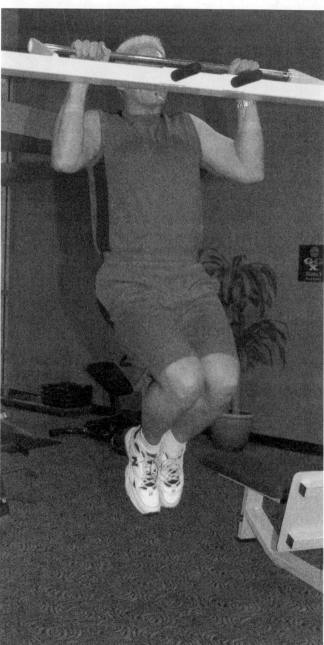

Pull-Ups

be done on a weight-assisted pull-up machine.

Sets and reps: *Weeks 1–2:* Two sets of 10 repetitions. *Weeks 3–7:* Three sets of maximum repetitions.

Tip: Try not to let your legs swing back and forth. If necessary, a spotter can hold your lower back to prevent swinging, or you can cross your feet to minimize swinging.

Twisting Sit-Ups

Body areas affected: Abdominal muscles and obliques.

Equipment needed: Exercise mat or flat, nonslippery surface.

Weight: Body weight.

Technique: Lie on your back with your hands crossed in front of your chest, your knees bent, and your feet flat on the floor. Raise yourself up and twist so that you touch your left knee with your right elbow. Lower yourself. Alternate with touching your right knee with your left elbow.

Sets and reps: Three sets of maximum repetitions.

Tip: Sit-ups may be harder on your lower back than crunches, and any twisting motion will have the same effect. Be extremely careful when doing this exercise if you have a lower back problem, and consult with your physician or physical therapist—who may tell you not to do it at all.

Lunge with Dumbbells or Barbells

Body areas affected: Quadriceps, glutes, and hamstrings.

Equipment needed: Dumbbells or barbell.

Weight: Body weight.

Technique: Stand erect with your feet shoulder-width apart. If you are using dumbbells, hold them at your sides with your palms turned toward your body. If you are using a barbell, hold it on your shoulders behind your head. (This requires a lot of practice, so it is probably best to use dumbbells at first.) Take one full step forward with your right leg so that your right foot is two feet in front of your left. Your weight should be evenly distributed. Lift your left heel, and move your left hip forward slightly into a pelvic tilt so that your left thigh is perpendicular to the floor. Hold that position, then slowly lower yourself until your left knee nearly touches the floor. Your lower body should be in contraction, including your abdomen, hamstrings, and quads. As you rise, concentrate on squeezing your legs together. Keep your feet in position.

Sets and reps: *Weeks 1–2:* Two sets of 12 repetitions. *Weeks 3–7:* Three sets of 12 repetitions. In the third set, add repetitions if you feel comfortable doing so.

Tips: Balance and posture are important in this exercise. Form becomes especially important; make sure that you have proper supervision for this exercise, particularly if you are using a barbell instead of dumbbells. Adding weight forces you to concentrate on balance, but it also helps to increase your strength more quickly.

Push-Ups (illustrated on p. 101)

Body areas affected: Pectorals, biceps, and triceps.

Equipment needed: Exercise/workout mat or flat, nonslippery surface.

Weight: Body weight.

Technique: Get into the standard push-up position, raised up on your arms with your legs extended and your feet together. Try not to lock your arms in this position. Slowly lower yourself until your nose is nearly touching the floor. Raise yourself back up by pushing with your arms. Keep your back flat throughout the exercise.

Sets and reps: Start with five push-ups, and each day try to do at least one more. If you get up to 15, try to do two sets of 10.

Tips: Go slowly—this will help you get the full benefit of the exercise. Changing the position of your hands—by positioning them farther apart or closer together, for example—will isolate a different part of your pectoral muscles.

Hip Roll (illustrated on p. 118)

Body areas affected: Abdominal muscles and obliques.

Equipment needed: Incline board or flat, nonslippery surface.

Weight: Body weight.

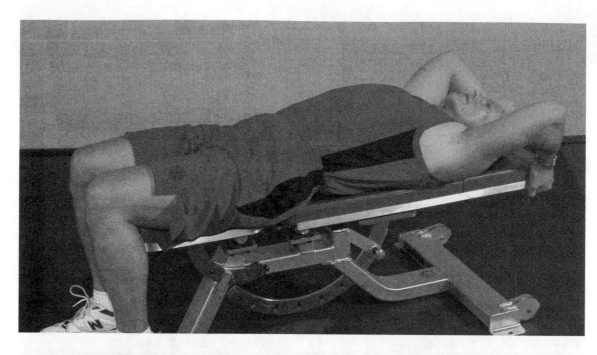

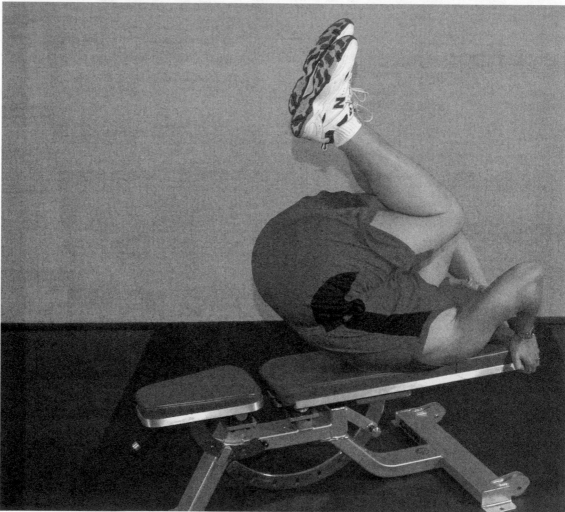

Hip Roll

Technique: This exercise is typically performed on a slant board of the type used for sit-ups. If you are using an incline board, lie on your back with your knees at the end of the board and your feet flat on the floor. Hold the head edge of the board with your hands. Roll your body up so that your knees approach your chest. Slowly bring them back down. If you are using a flat surface, lie on your back and perform the motion just described.

Sets and reps: Weeks 1–2: Three sets of 12 repetitions. *Weeks 3–4:* Three sets of 15 repetitions. *Weeks 5–6:* Three sets of 17 repetitions. *Week 7:* Three sets of 20 repetitions. In the third set, add repetitions if you feel comfortable doing so.

Tip: Keep your lower back as flat as possible on the surface while you are doing this exercise—don't arch it.

Seated Leg Curl (illustrated on pp. 92–93)

Body area affected: Hamstrings.

Equipment needed: Leg curl machine.

Technique: Sit with your back flush against the padded back support and your calves on top of the leg pads. Use a seatbelt if one is available. Start with your legs extended and slowly flex them while holding on to the side bars. Hold and contract, then slowly bring your legs back up to the starting position.

Sets and reps: Weeks 1–2: Two sets of 12 repetitions. *Weeks 3–4:* Two sets of 10 repetitions. *Weeks 5–7:* Two sets of 8 repetitions. In the third set, add repetitions if you feel comfortable doing so.

Tip: Don't arch your back.

Preacher Curl (illustrated on p. 120)

Body area affected: Biceps.

Equipment needed: Preacher bench and dumbbells, barbell, or EZ curl bar, or preacher curl machine.

Technique: Rest your elbows and forearms on the preacher stand and fully extend your arms. Grasp the barbell or dumbbells with an underhand grip. Curl the weight as you would in the Biceps Curl until the bar almost touches your collarbone. Slowly return the barbell or dumbbells to the starting position.

Sets and reps: Weeks 1–2: Three sets of 10 repetitions. *Weeks 3–5:* Three sets of eight repetitions. *Weeks 6–7:* Three sets of 12 repetitions; in the third set, add repetitions if you feel comfortable doing so.

Tip: Use light weight initially, since the design of the machine makes it difficult to cheat and use muscles other than your biceps.

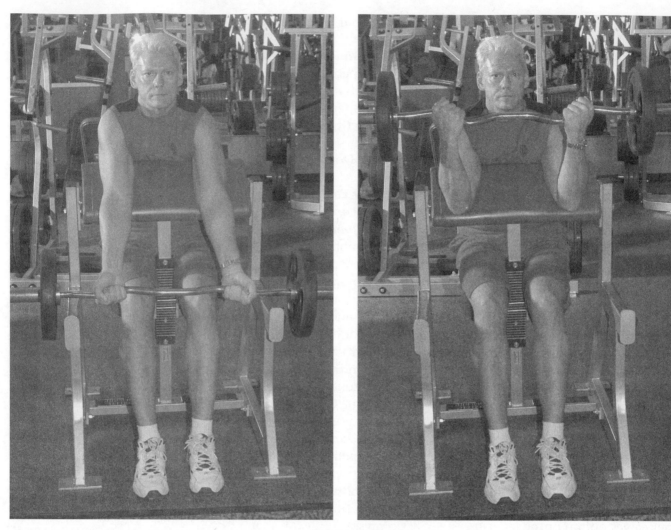

Preacher Curl

9

Supplementary Exercises

This chapter contains exercises that you may want to progress to after you have mastered the exercises in the sample men's and women's programs in Chapter 8. Some of these new exercises are more difficult to master and will force you to concentrate even more on technique. To avoid injury, they need to be learned under the supervision of trained gym personnel.

As with any new exercise, start with very light weight when you are learning these exercises—perhaps even lighter than you think you can handle. It is often advisable to use a barbell with no weight plates to practice the motion of a new barbell exercise. When you feel comfortable with the exercise, add weight, but do so gradually.

CHEST

Incline Bench Press
This exercise works your lower and upper pecs more than your middle pecs; you will feel the stress in those areas. Since it is easy to do this exercise incorrectly, be sure to have your technique

approved by trained gym personnel. You can use either dumbbells or a very light barbell. Use a bench that has an incline of between 45 and 70 degrees. Bring the weight down over your chest, not over your shoulders, when you are lowering it.

Pullovers (Straight Arm and Bent Arm)
Pullovers can be done with your arms straight or bent. Lie with your feet on the floor and your head slightly beyond the end of the bench. Use very light weight initially, and hold the bar with an overhand grip above your chest. Slowly bring the bar over your head until it is directly behind your head. Don't arch your back as you pull the weight over your head; you can avoid arching your back by putting your heels on the bench with your knees bent.

Push-Ups with Feet on Balance Ball/ Medicine Ball
This challenging exercise forces you to use your trunk to balance your body while you are using your chest and shoulders to perform the push-up. Try it with your knees on the ball,

then with your feet; the latter is more difficult.

Push-Ups with Hands on Balance Ball
This exercise is easier to do than a standard push-up and tests your balance more than it works your body. It is a good introduction to push-ups for people who are overweight.

SHOULDERS

Bent-Over Lateral Raise
This exercise is similar to the regular lateral raise, but it works a different area of your deltoid muscles. Since it requires practice to do this raise

correctly, use a mirror to check your technique. With dumbbells at your side, bend at the waist, keeping your back flat (so that you don't hyperextend your lower back). Your head should be gently lifted, but not out of alignment with your spine. Use the same motion as you would for a lateral raise, with bowed elbows. Concentrate on lifting with your shoulder, as opposed to your shoulder blades; if you are hunching your shoulder blades up and down, you are doing the exercise incorrectly.

Rotator Cuff Exercises
Dumbbell Rotation (Seated)
Sit on a bench or other surface, with your back straight. Hold a dumbbell

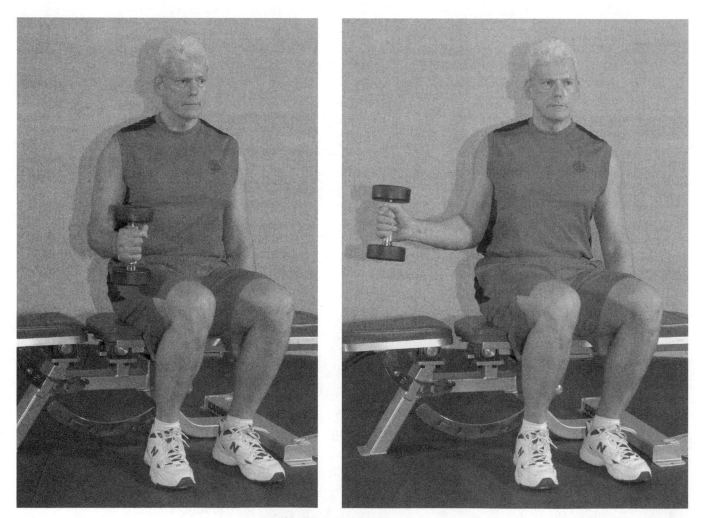

Dumbbell Rotation (Seated)

in one hand and keep your elbow close to your side and bent 90 degrees. Rotate your arm away from your body, then back to the starting position.

Dumbbell Rotation (Prone)

(illustrated on p. 124)

Lie on your side, with your head resting on one hand and holding a dumbbell in the opposite hand. Keep your elbow close to your side and bent 90 degrees. Starting with the dumbbell away from your body, slowly bring it back toward your chest, then raise it back to the starting position.

Empty Can

Stand erect, holding a dumbbell in each hand. Raise your arms to about shoulder height and extend them in front of you at an angle about 30 degrees away from your body. Rotate your hands so your palms are turned toward the floor, then slowly make a repetitive motion as if the dumbbells were two cans and you are emptying liquid from them.

Dead Lift with Hex Bar or Universal Machine

A hex bar is a bar constructed in a hexagonal shape so that you can stand inside it and grip the handles on the sides; weights are placed on the bar at either side. Stand with your feet about shoulder-width apart, grip the handles of the hex bar, and squat down, keeping your back straight (this is important!) and your head forward. Slowly straighten your legs as you pull the bar up past your knees until you are back to a standing position. Return the weight to the floor while bending your knees slowly and keeping your back straight.

This exercise can be simulated on a Universal weight machine using the bench press. Remove the bench, stand on top of a box, facing the bar that is low enough so that you have to squat down to reach it. Perform the exercise as described above.

ARMS

Reverse Curl

The Reverse Curl is like the Biceps Curl except that you use an overhand grip; the exercise works your forearms in addition to your biceps. Since the motion is somewhat unnatural, make sure that you are doing it correctly, and don't overgrip the dumbbell or barbell. If you are using a barbell, start with light weight and grip the bar closer than you would for the Biceps Curl, with your thumbs about one to three inches apart. With the bar resting on your thighs, flex your wrist first, then pull the bar up. Relax on the way down, and repeat. Focus on not pushing with your hips. Throughout the exercise, try to relax your wrists to avoid straining them.

French Curl

You use an EZ curl barbell, which is not as wide as a regular barbell and has a dip in the middle where you grip it. Start with very light weight. Sitting in a chair with a back support, start with the weight directly above your head and your arms slightly bowed. Slowly bend your arms at the elbows and move the weight behind your head, then raise it back to the starting position. The key is to make sure that your upper arms remain parallel to the floor. Don't bow your arms back or let your shoulder blades move back. A mirror allows you to check that your arms are at the correct angle.)

Wrist Curl

Sit with your arms resting on your thighs and your hands extended past your knees. Using a barbell or dumbbells, lower the weight as far as you can by only bending your wrists, then

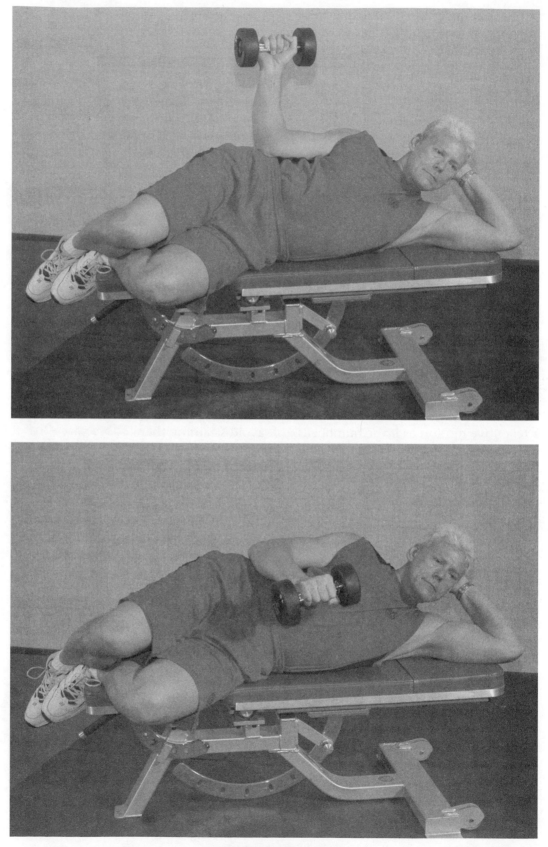

Dumbbell Rotation (Prone)

raise it back to the starting position. Do this exercise with your hands in both underhand and overhand grips.

Another exercise that strengthens your wrists and forearms is the Lateral Wrist Curl, in which you use a dumbbell with a weight attached to one end. With one hand, hold the dumbbell in the middle with the weight facing up, rotate the bar to the side, and then back to the upright position.

Wrist Roller

This simple exercise can be performed using the wrist station on a Universal machine or by using a wrist roller you make yourself. For the latter, tie a length of rope to the middle of a piece of wood or metal that approximates a small barbell in size and shape, and tie a weight to the other end of the rope. Simply roll the bar in your hands using an overhand grip, winding the rope around the bar as the weight is raised up.

UPPER BACK

Bent-Over Row

This exercise can be performed using a barbell or the low pulley station on a Universal machine. Stand with your feet shoulder-width apart and your elbows and knees slightly bent, holding the bar with an overhand grip. Keeping your back straight, bend over and lower the weight. Raise the weight back up to your chest in this bent-over position, then lower it back down.

Chin-Ups

Chin-ups are excellent for building your biceps. The motion is the same as that for a pull-up, except that your hands are in an underhand grip. You should be able to do more repetitions with chin-ups, since they are easier to do than pull-ups.

LOWER BACK

Spine Extension

This exercise strengthens your lower back muscles, which helps stabilize your spine. Most important, spine extensions use only your body weight for resistance. Get on your hands and knees on the floor, with your back straight and your face toward the floor. With one smooth motion, lift your left arm and extend it fully in front of you while extending your left leg behind you with your toe pointed. You should be able to draw a more or less straight line from the tip of your fingers to the tips of your toes. Repeat with your right arm and leg. You can also do this exercise alternating arms and legs (lifting your left arm and right leg simultaneously, for instance).

To make sure that your back is flat during this exercise, have someone put a broomstick on your back; if it rolls off, your back isn't flat enough.

Good Morning

Use very light weight and proceed slowly as you learn this exercise, which can place great stress on your lower back. Stand erect, with your feet shoulder-width apart and your knees slightly bent. Hold a barbell on your shoulders behind your head. In one fluid motion, bend forward at the waist while keeping your head upright, then return to the starting position.

ABDOMINALS AND OBLIQUES

Isometric Abdominal Exercise

This exercise can be done anywhere, anytime, and with no equipment at all. Tighten your abdominal muscles and hold them that way for about 20 or 30 seconds—that's it! Remember to breathe while you are doing the exercise.

Reverse Beetle

This exercise can be done with only a bench or table. Sit on the bench so that your knees are just over the edge. Lean backward a little and hold onto the sides of the bench with your hands. Bring your knees up toward your chest—not all the way, but so that your thighs form about a 90-degree angle with your upper body. Then extend them out in front of you until they are almost straight.

Modified Abdominal Crunch

Lie on your back as if you were about to do a regular abdominal crunch. Let your knees fall to one side while keeping your back flat on the floor, and do the crunch from that position. If you have a lower back problem, be particularly careful when attempting this exercise.

Standing Isolated Rib Cage Motion

Stand erect, with your back straight, your feet shoulder-width apart, and your knees slightly bent. Without twisting your hips, lift your rib cage up and over to the right, then bring it back to the center. If you keep your hips stationary, you should feel tightness in your obliques ("love handles"). Use a mirror to make sure that you are doing this exercise correctly.

10

Alternative Training

One of the biggest obstacles to staying in shape is finding the time to exercise. Fitting a workout into your busy schedule can be more challenging than the workout itself.

Fortunately, there are many exercises that you can do on your own, either at home or on the road. These exercises don't require expensive equipment or fancy gadgets (see Chapter 12 for a description of different types of home fitness equipment). Some of these exercises simulate exercises that you can do in the gym. They aren't a true substitute for a full workout in the gym, of course, but they certainly can help you keep your muscles and joints limber and active.

For instance, you can do a wide variety of upper and lower body exercises using a stretch cord or exercise band that approximate exercises in a gym, from Hip Abduction to Leg Curl and from Triceps Extension to Biceps Curl. This equipment is lightweight and can be packed for easy transport when you are traveling.

For some of the exercises in this chapter, you will need the following pieces of equipment, all of which are relatively inexpensive and easy to find at your local gym or sporting goods store. Some are items that you may even have around the house.

- Soft foam ball
- A stretch cord (also called a weight band), with a loop or handle at each end
- A rubber exercise band (similar to a stretch cord but made of thin, flat rubber)
- A balance board (or a circular piece of plywood at least three quarters of an inch thick)
- A rubber ball, about the size of a softball
- A small dumbbell (one to four pounds)
- An exercise mat (about 2 feet wide and 6 feet long)
- A jump rope
- A balance ball
- Ankle and wrist weights

Abdominal Crunch with Exercise Band

Lie on the floor, with your knees bent and your feet flat on the floor. Loop the exercise band around your ankles and, with your feet together and your knees bent, raise your legs off the floor. Hold the exercise band on the floor with your hands so there is no slack. From this position, lift your upper body off the floor as you would for a regular crunch.

Leg Lift

Lie on the floor, with one leg straight in front of you and the other bent at the knee. Slowly raise your straightened leg as high as you can. Hold for 10 seconds. Repeat five to 10 times.

Squeezing Ball

Hold a soft foam ball in your hand, with your palm upward. Squeeze the ball 15 to 20 times.

Stretch Cord Pulling

Use a length of stretch cord about four feet long. Place one end on the other side of a door and close the door securely (or loop one end of the cord around your foot and extend your leg so the cord is taut). Flexing your wrist, pull the other end of the cord with your hand until you feel moderate resistance. Repeat 10 to 15 times.

Prone Hip Extension

Lie face down on a flat, firm surface. Raise one leg from the hip to a count of four, then slowly lower it to a count of eight. Do three sets of 10, then repeat with your other leg.

Standing Rubber Band Flexion and Abduction

Tie a rubber exercise band around a fixed object such as a banister. Wrap the band around one of your ankles. Flex your leg from the hip against the resistance of the rubber band. Extend your leg to a count of four, and flex it to a count of eight. Do three sets of 10, then repeat with your other leg.

Standing Rubber Band Hip Extension

Tie a rubber exercise band around a fixed object such as a banister. Wrap the band around one of your ankles. Extend and lower your leg from the hip against the resistance of the rubber band. Extend your leg to a count of four, and flex it to a count of eight. Do three sets of 10, then repeat with your other leg.

Abductor Raise

Lie on your side, with your head resting on one hand. Bend your leg on the floor and keep the other leg straight. Slowly lift the straight leg, hold it up for five seconds, then lower it. Repeat 20 to 30 times, then repeat with your other leg. (Ankle weights may be used to increase effectiveness.)

Quadriceps Leg Raise

Sit in a semirecumbent position, leaning on your hands behind you. With one knee bent, squeeze the quadriceps of the opposite, straight leg and raise it 45 degrees. Hold 10 to 20 seconds, then lower the leg. Repeat eight to 10 times, then repeat with your other leg.

Quadriceps Knee Extension

(illustrated on p. 130)

Sit on a chair, with your knees bent and your feet on the floor. Straighten and extend one leg slowly, then lower it back down slowly. (Use ankle weights to increase effectiveness.) Repeat 20 to 30 times, then repeat with your other leg.

Step-Ups

Stand in front of a bench or a double-step two feet high. Step up onto the bench, straighten your knees fully, and then step down. Repeat at a steady pace. Once you feel comfortable with the motion, add weights to your hands.

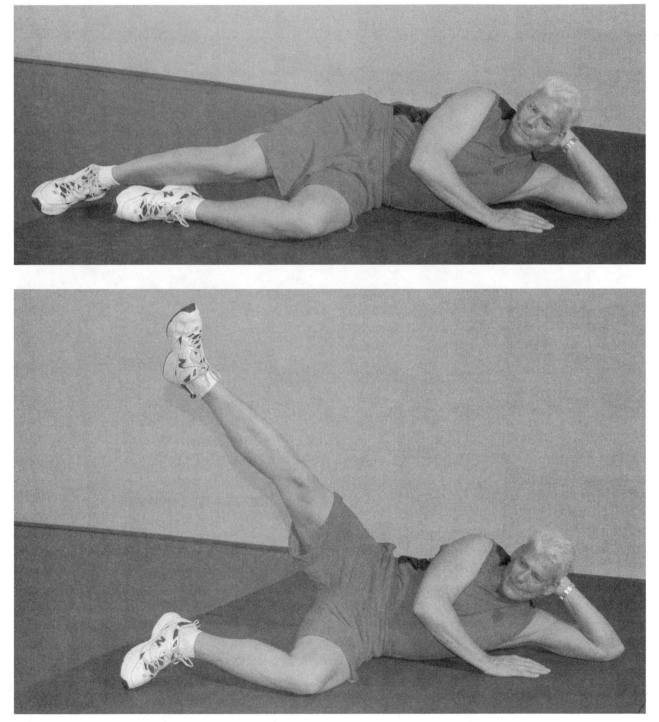

Abductor Raise

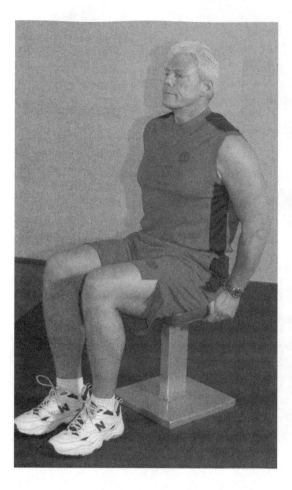
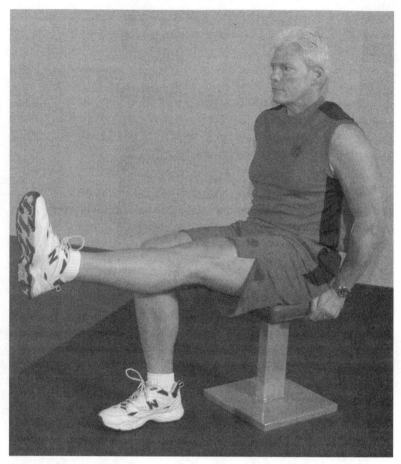

Quadriceps Knee Extension

Hamstring Curl

Stand with your thighs against a flat surface such as a wall. Bend one knee as far as it can go, hold for ten seconds, then lower the foot slowly. Use ankle weights or a stretch cord to increase effectiveness. Repeat 20 to 30 times, then repeat with your other leg.

Stretch Cord Inversion

Use a length of stretch cord about four feet long. Loop one end around a stationary object and sit on a chair with your right side toward the stationary object. Cross your right leg over your left. Loop the free end of the stretch cord around the ball of your right foot. Position yourself so that the cord has moderate tension. Rotate your right foot inward, so that the cord is pulled tighter and you feel moderate resistance. Hold for 10 to 15 seconds, then relax. Repeat 10 to 15 times, then repeat with your left foot.

Stretch Cord Eversion

Use a length of stretch cord about four feet long. Loop one end around a stationary object and sit on a chair with your right side toward the stationary object. Cross your left leg over your right. Loop the free end of the stretch cord around the outside of your left foot. Position yourself so that the cord has moderate tension. Rotate your right foot outward, so that the cord is pulled tighter and you feel moderate resistance. Hold for 10 to 15 seconds, then relax. Repeat 10 to 15 times, then repeat with your right foot.

Stretch Cord Extension

Use a length of stretch cord about four feet long. Loop one end around a stationary object and sit on a chair facing the stationary object. Cross your right leg over your left. Loop the free end of the cord over the top of your right foot. Position yourself so that the cord has moderate tension. Extend your ankle back, toward your head, against the resistance. Hold for 10 to 15 seconds, then relax. Repeat 10 to 15 times, then repeat with your left foot.

Toe Raise

Stand with the balls of your feet and your toes on a thick book (such as a telephone book). Holding onto a support, slowly lower your heels to the floor, then slowly raise your heels as high as you can. Hold for 8 to 10 seconds. Repeat 15 to 20 times.

Toe Scrunch

Place a cloth or towel on the floor near a chair. Sit on the chair and place the toes of one foot on the cloth. Keeping your heel flat on the floor, use your toes to scrunch up the cloth. Repeat 10 to 20 times, then repeat with your other foot.

Walking on Heels

While standing, lift your toes off the floor. Start walking on just your heels. Take 10 to 20 steps.

Squats (illustrated on pp. 132–133)

Stand erect, with your feet shoulder-width apart and your arms extended straight out. Keeping your heels on the floor and your knees over your feet, squat down slowly, then return to a standing position. Keep your back as straight as possible. Repeat 20 to 30 times. If necessary, place your hands on an object like a table or chair back for balance.

Saucers and Balance Boards

(saucers illustrated on pp. 134–136)

Saucers and balance boards are great devices for stretching and strengthening your ankles, as well as improving balance.

Saucers, usually made of plastic or rubber and about the size of dinner plates, can add a new twist to movements like squats or lunges by forcing you to concentrate on balance and stability while you perform specific exercises. Ask your trainer or fitness professional about ways to incorporate saucers into your workouts.

Balance boards—also called wobble, or rocker, boards—come in different sizes and can be set at different angles. They operate on the same principle as saucers, with a flat surface (square or round) attached to a round base that rolls with your movements. They improve balance and coordination, as well as trunk and pelvic strength. Begin moving, at first slowly, then start pivoting and making sharper movements as you feel more comfortable.

Butt Kicks

Run in place, swinging your arms in a controlled motion. Kick your legs back up behind you so that your heels lightly touch your buttocks.

Regular Dips

This exercise is normally done using parallel bars in a gym, but you can use two stationary objects with flat surfaces about waist high. Place one hand on each surface and lift yourself up until your arms are straight. With your knees bent, lower yourself slowly by flexing your arms. Lift yourself back up by extending your arms. Cross your feet to keep your legs from separating.

Text continues on p. 137.

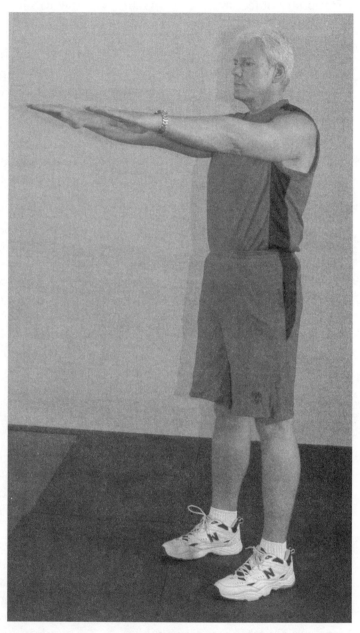

Squats . . .

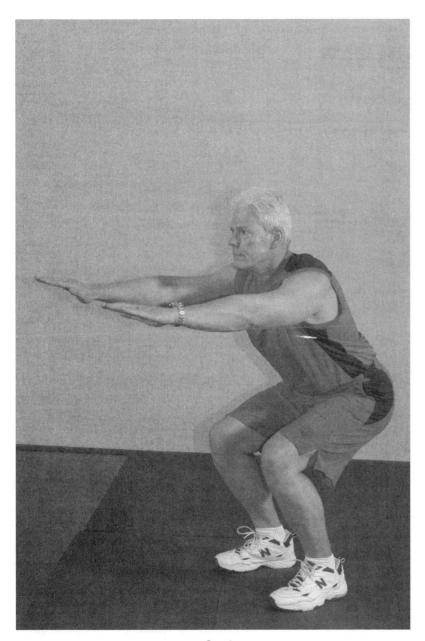

... Squats

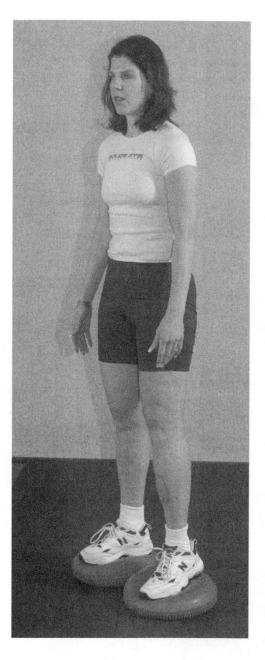
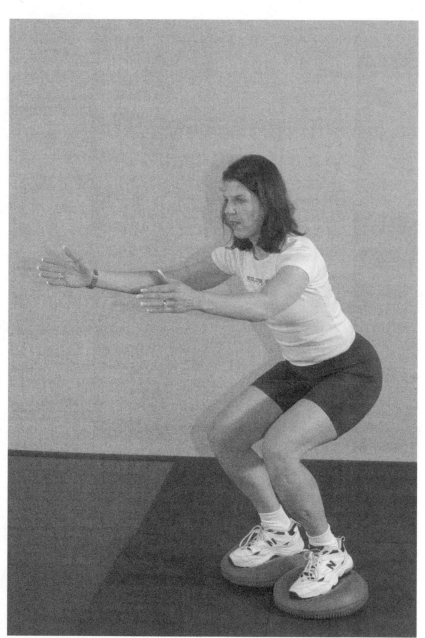

Saucers

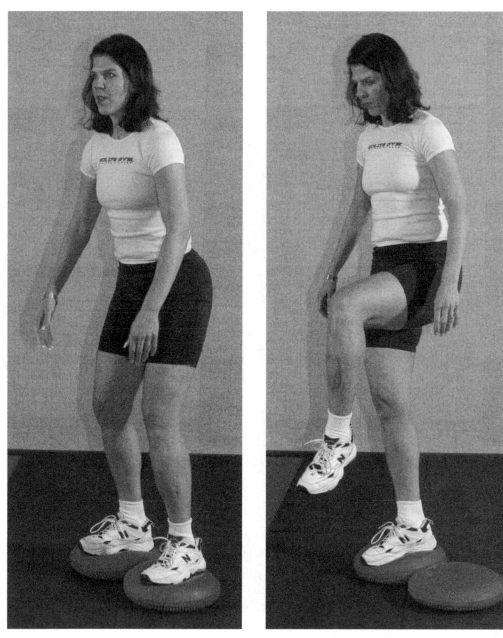

Saucers

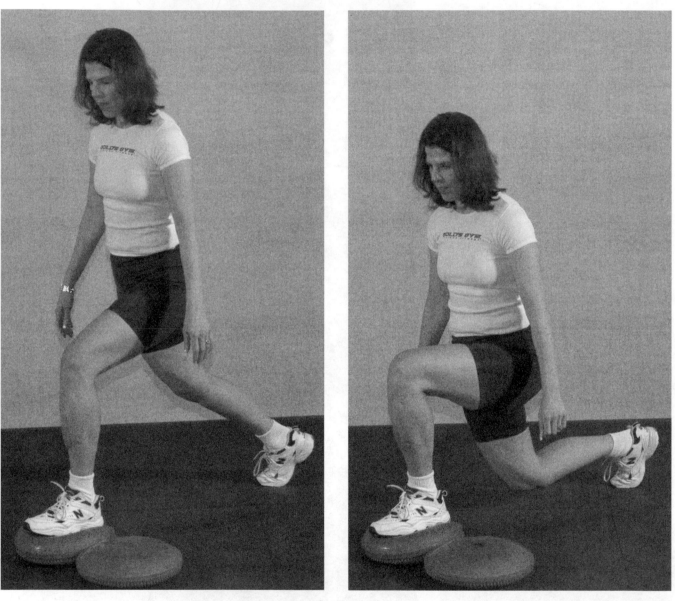

Saucers

Modified Dips

Place two benches parallel to each other, about three or four feet apart. With your feet on one bench and your hands on the other, lower and raise your body with your arms.

Arm Swings

Stand erect with your feet shoulder-width apart and holding a one- or two-pound weight in each hand. Swing your arms back and forth as if you were running. Concentrate on good form and controlling your swings.

High Knees

Run in place, swinging your arms in a controlled manner as you are running. Lift your knees high off the ground, being sure to land on your toes or on the balls of your feet. Concentrate on balance, and get into a rhythm by doing a small bounce or hop on each step.

Push-Ups to T Stance

Perform a regular push-up, but as you extend your arms and raise up, rotate your body and raise one arm

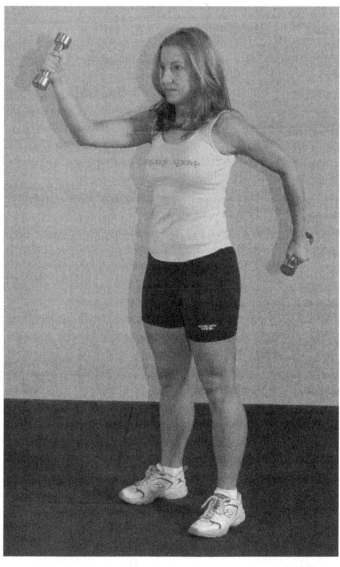
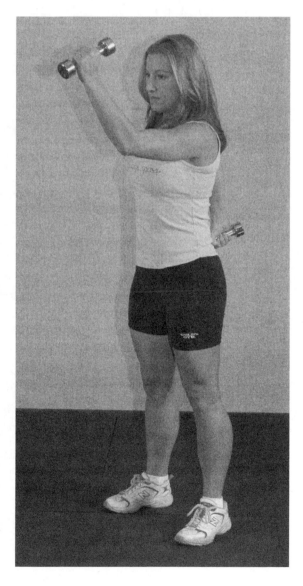

Arm Swings

upward, balancing yourself on the other arm so your arms form a T with your body. Bring your arm back down to the floor and repeat with the other arm.

Squat Thrusts

Stand with your feet together and your hands at your sides. In one continuous motion, squat down, steadying yourself with your hands on the floor, then extend your legs behind so that you are in a push-up position. Bring your legs back up

underneath you as they were, then stand upright.

Jumping Rope

You can burn up to 200 calories in as little as 15 minutes by jumping rope. Choose a rope that is long enough for you; people of average height (5-foot-4 to 5-foot-10) should use a nine-foot rope, and taller people should use a 10-foot rope. You can alternate legs, jump off both legs simultaneously, or do any variations you choose. Make sure that the ceiling is high enough!

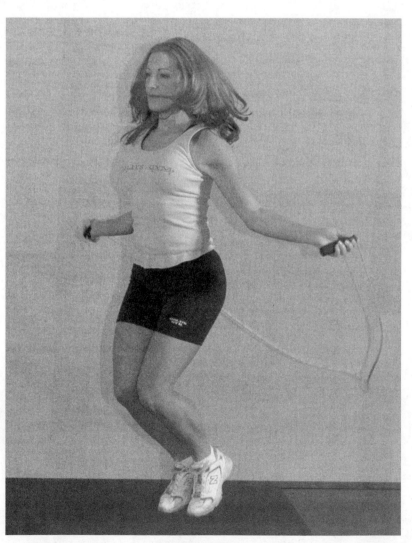

Jumping Rope

11

Nutrition

Everyone needs to eat right, but it is especially important for people who exercise regularly and push their bodies to the limits of fatigue and endurance, and therefore need to replace depleted stores of energy. Some athletes use supplements and other products to enhance their training. These will be addressed later in this chapter, but a healthy, balanced diet and a good workout plan are more than sufficient to keep you fit and performing at your best. A healthy diet for an athlete is also a healthy basic diet: the proper balance of protein, carbohydrates, and fat.

Eating right is not an easy task— not with so many bad options available (like fast food, sweets, and juice drinks that are mostly corn syrup). Working out regularly, however, almost forces you to eat right. If you don't, you'll notice it fairly soon, because you'll feel sluggish and unmotivated.

THE BUILDING BLOCKS OF NUTRITION

Understanding what foods you need in your diet requires an understanding of the nutritional components contained in those foods and what they do for your body.

Water

Water helps maintain your body temperature, transport nutrients, and flush toxins from your body. Although it is absolutely essential to stay hydrated when you are exercising, as discussed earlier in this book, you need water even if you are not active.

Protein

Protein helps your body's tissues grow and heal. It also supplies amino acids, assists in the formation of hormones and enzymes, and aids the development of antibodies. It is generally recommended that you get 20% to 30% of your daily calories from protein.

Carbohydrates

There are two types of carbohydrates: simple and complex. Simple carbohydrates include refined sugars (like white sugar) and sugars that occur naturally (like those found in fruit). Complex carbohydrates occur in breads, pasta, and vegetables, and are very valuable to your body.

When your body digests food, it is broken down into substances that the body can use. Carbohydrates become glucose molecules that enter the bloodstream and feed your muscles, organs, and brain.

Fat

People tend to be wary of fat, but it plays a vital nutritional role. Fat insulates your body, protects nerve pathways and organs, and provides a vehicle for fat-soluble vitamins. You need fat in your diet, but you also need to be careful about how much you ingest, as well as what type.

Fats are classified as saturated or unsaturated. Saturated fats are solid at room temperature, like lard. They can be harmful to arteries by causing blockages. Unsaturated fats do not pack together as tightly, and therefore they cause fewer blockages. The best unsaturated fats are found in foods like olives, peanuts, and walnuts.

It is generally recommended that you get between 20% and 30% of your daily calories from fat. Unfortunately, the average American gets 37% of his or her calories from fat. Your diet should emphasize foods that have healthier, unsaturated fats as much as possible.

Vitamins and Minerals

Vitamins regulate biochemical reactions in your body. They assist your body in digesting and using nutrients from other sources. Vitamins can be either fat-soluble or water-soluble. The body stores vitamins that are fat-soluble, so you can build up too many of them if you take them in large quantities. When you take an excessive quantity of a water-soluble vitamin, your body simply flushes out the excess in urine. A daily multivitamin pill from your

pharmacy can supplement the vitamins in the food you eat.

Minerals help carry nerve signals, build bones, and clot blood. Most people do not need mineral supplements, although many women suffer from iron deficiency and need to augment their diet with iron supplements (see the section "Iron and Calcium" below).

BALANCE AND MODERATION

If you are training intensively or engaged in competition, you are expending more energy and thus require more nutrients for refueling. This should not be an excuse to overeat, however. The amount of food you eat should be in proportion to the amount of energy you expend. When you achieve that balance, it is easy to maintain your weight at a healthy level. Here are some tips:

- Keep your food portions modest. When you have a smaller amount of food on your plate, you will find it easier to eat in moderation.
- As much as possible, eat at regular times every day. Skipping meals or eating too much between meals is detrimental to a balanced diet. When you skip meals, you may become extremely hungry, which can lead to gorging.
- Eat plenty of vegetables, fruits, and grain products. Most Americans do not eat enough of these foods. Keep fresh fruits and vegetables in your home—and reach for them when you want a snack.
- Avoid eating a lot of fried foods, creamy sauces, butter, red meat, and other high-fat foods. Eat skim or low-fat dairy products and lean cuts of meat instead. On the other hand,

do not deny yourself all your favorite foods. The key is moderation: Eat them in small portions and relatively infrequently.

- Eat sugar in moderation, and eat moderate amounts of salt and sodium-rich foods.
- If you drink alcoholic beverages, do so in moderation.
- Eat a variety of foods that are high in fiber. Fiber plays a critical role in your health. Eat fruits with their skins, and eat whole-grain breads and cereals.
- Drink a lot of water. Every adult needs at least eight 8-ounce glasses of water a day. If you are physically active, you should drink even more water.

NUTRITION GUIDELINES FOR ATHLETES

Carbohydrate Requirements

Carbohydrates are the nutrient of choice for athletes. The brain, muscles, and red blood cells rely primarily on carbohydrates for their major source of energy. Anaerobic activities such as weight lifting and sprinting use only carbohydrates as an energy source.

Eating whole-grain foods, fruits, and vegetables will help you meet your daily requirement of carbohydrates. You should avoid simple and processed carbohydrates, such as white flour, processed foods, simple sugars, and alcohol.

The following guidelines reflect the energy expenditure of someone in moderate to heavy training. It may be necessary to decrease the amount of carbohydrates consumed if your activity level is lower.

How Much Carbohydrate Do You Need?

Ideally, you should get 60% to 70% of your total calories from carbo-hydrates, or about six to 10 grams of carbohydrate per kilogram of body weight. (To calculate your weight in kilograms, divide your body weight in pounds by 2.2.)

Foods high in carbohydrates include the following:

	GRAMS
Applesauce (1 cup)	60
Bagel (1 large)	60
Banana (1 large)	60
Boost® energy drink (8 oz.)	45
Cereal (1 cup)	24
Nachos (1 serving)	31
Pasta (1 cup)	34
Pizza (1 slice)	21
Potato (1 large)	60
Power Bar® nutrition bar	45
Rice (1 cup)	50
Turkey sandwich	35

You should read product labels to find out the carbohydrate content of the foods you buy. For nonlabeled foods, the following table can help you determine carbohydrate content in general terms:

	GRAMS
Bread (1 slice)	15
Vegetable (½ cup)	5
Salad greens (1 cup)	5
Fruit (1 small)	15
Dairy product (1 cup)	12

Pre-Workout or Pre-Game Meals

Eating properly before you work out or compete can be just as important as warming up or cooling down. A good rule of thumb is to eat three to four hours prior to your workout or competition; this will give your body time to digest and absorb nutrients. Ideally, the meal should contain the following:

- Lean protein
- High-carbohydrate foods
- A small amount of fat
- Plenty of fluids

Some athletes prefer to use liquid meal replacements instead of solid food prior to a workout or competition. This is an acceptable alternative and can be improved with the addition of fresh fruit. Liquid meal replacements, which leave your stomach more quickly than solid foods, require less time for digestion and absorption of nutrients.

Refueling During Exercise

You should consume 30 to 60 grams of carbohydrates per hour. Sports drinks usually contain about 14 grams per eight ounces. Water will keep you hydrated, but sports drinks will keep you going better and longer.

Refueling After Exercise

You need to consume carbohydrates after exercise to replace glycogen stores (carbohydrates stored in the muscle and liver) that have been depleted. Proper replacement can be achieved by consuming about 1 to 1.5 grams of carbohydrates per kilogram of body weight within five to 30 minutes after exercising, and 100 grams per hour for one to two hours thereafter. Research also indicates that the addition of protein at this time aids in glycogen replacement.

A good way to achieve this glycogen replacement is to drink a carbohydrate beverage before leaving the gym and eat carbohydrates at lunch (assuming you worked out in the morning) or on the way home from the gym. This can be easily done by consuming a normal meal that includes high-carbohydrate items, such as breads, pasta, fruit, and fruit juices.

Protein Requirements

Athletes have an increased need for protein because of their training and physical activity. You should consume between 1.2 and 1.8 grams of protein per kilogram of body weight. The following table indicates the amount of protein in some common foods:

	GRAMS
Boost® energy drink (8 oz.)	10
Burger (4 oz.)	28
Cheese (1.5 oz.—the size of 4 dice)	8
Chicken (4 oz.)	28
Egg, whole	7
Egg white	3.5
Meat (1 oz. of chicken, fish, or turkey)	7
Milk (1 cup)	8
Nuts (¼ cup)	7
Pasta (1 cup)	6
Peanut butter (2 teaspoons)	8
Pizza (1 slice)	16
Power Bar® Protein Plus	24
Tuna (1 can)	28
Yogurt (1 cup)	8-9

Some Tips About Protein

- Although protein is important for the athlete, it cannot provide energy by itself. If carbohydrates are restricted, the body uses protein as an energy source, which depletes the amount of protein available for muscle synthesis. The key is to balance your protein and carbohydrate intake.
- Protein consumed in excess of what your body needs will be stored as fat.
- High-protein diets require additional water to eliminate the nitrogen component of protein. If you don't drink extra water, dehydration can occur.
- Your body processes protein from food better than protein from amino acid supplements.
- Too much protein can lead to calcium loss through urine.
- Choose lean, high-quality protein foods such as chicken, fish, turkey, egg whites, and lean meats, such as pork loin, London broil, and

sirloin cuts. Avoid cuts of meat from the rib portion of an animal.

- Whey and soy protein drinks are acceptable as long as they are part of a balanced diet, since they may lack several vital nutrients.

Sample High-Protein, Adequate-Carbohydrate Diet

The following sample diet contains about 33% protein, 50% carbohydrates, and 20% fat.

Breakfast
Omelet (6-8 egg whites)
Toast (2 slices whole wheat, with
    2 tablespoons butter/margarine)
Fruit (1, or fruit juice)

Post-workout
Boost® energy drink (8 oz.)
Gatorade® (1 bottle)

Lunch
Salad (large tossed, with light dressing)
Chicken, fish, or turkey (8 oz., on a roll
    or with 2 slices of bread)
Fruit (1 fresh)

Snack
Protein bar

Dinner
Chicken, fish, or turkey (12 oz.)
Pasta, noodles, or rice (1 cup)
Greens (unlimited)
Butter/margarine (2 tablespoons)
Fruit (1)

Fat Requirements

The primary function of fat is to provide energy. However, a diet high in fat can be detrimental to your athletic performance and overall health. Athletes should strive for a diet that has 20% to 30% fat. A diet consisting of less than 20% fat can lower testosterone levels, especially after resistance exercises such as weight lifting. Your diet should emphasize fats in the good, better, and great categories below:

Saturated fats (not so good)
Butter, hydrogenated oils, lard,
    red meat, egg yolks, and chicken
    skin

Polyunsaturated fats (good)
Corn oil, soybean oil, and safflower
    oil

Monounsaturated fats (better)
Olive oil, peanut oil, canola oil,
    and nuts

Omega-3 fatty acids (great)
Salmon, walnuts, canola oil, and
    flaxseed

Foods high in fat include butter, margarine, gravy, fried foods, red meat, cookies, fries, salad dressings, and snack foods.

Vitamin Requirements

High therapeutic doses of vitamins do not improve athletic performance. However, if a diet is lacking in vitamins, a supplement can improve the nutritional status of an athlete. A multivitamin supplement of 100% of the RDA is recommended for all individuals.

Research has indicated that athletes may benefit from the addition of certain antioxidant nutrients. These vitamins have been associated with decreased recovery time and decreased muscle soreness. They include vitamins C and E, as well as selenium. The best way to obtain these nutrients is to include the following in your diet:

- Whole-grain foods
- Lean cuts of meat
- Nuts and seeds
- Fruits and vegetables (including at least 1 citrus fruit per day)

When choosing a supplement, look for the USP marking on the package. This ensures that the product has met the U.S. Pharmacopeia's standards for quality, purity, and potency.

Fluid Requirements

Dehydration by as little as 1% of your body weight can cause a decrease in performance. Athletes need to consume a minimum of two to five quarts of fluid every day in order to stay properly hydrated. Follow these guidelines to maintain proper hydration:

	OUNCES
Wake-up time or two hours before exercise	16
15 minutes before exercise	4-8
During exercise (every 15 minutes)	6-12
After exercise (for each pound of fluid lost)	16-24

Avoid fluids with high caffeine content, such as coffee, tea, and colas. If you do consume these beverages, you must consume an additional eight ounces of water for each eight-ounce serving to combat the diuretic effect of caffeine.

DIETARY SUPPLEMENTS

Striving to be "the best one can be" is characteristic of athletes at all levels, from the beginner to the Olympic champion. Unfortunately, the desire of athletes to gain an edge on their competition has led to an explosion in the number of nutritional supplements that claim to improve athletic performance. Laws allow manufacturers of these supplements to make claims, mostly unproved, about the effects of their products as long as they do not claim to treat or cure a specific disease. The result is that the marketplace has become overloaded with products that are harmless at best and may contain the potential for harm if they are abused or taken by people who should not be taking them for medical reasons.

First, it is important to differentiate between a drug and a supplement. The former is a substance that has been approved by the Food and Drug Administration (FDA) as having a specific effect on the body, whether to change the body's structure or function or to treat disease. Dietary supplements, on the other hand, do not have to be FDA-approved, since they are not classified as drugs, and they may not have any nutritional value at all.

Credible scientific evidence for the benefits of dietary supplements is lacking. A well-balanced diet that addresses the need for appropriate levels of protein, carbohydrates, and fat will enable you to meet your athletic goals.

Iron and Calcium

Iron and calcium deficiencies are common among women and should be addressed when embarking on a weight training program. Low levels of iron can lead to fatigue and decreased performance, as well as to anemia. To avoid this, eat foods that are rich in iron, such as meat, chicken, and fish. At the same time, be sure to consume citrus fruits and juices, since citrus aids your body's absorption of iron. Do not take iron supplements without consulting your physician, since too much iron can be dangerous to your health.

Many women do not get enough calcium in their daily diet. This deficiency can be exacerbated by intense training, which can lead to irregular menstrual cycles and decreased bone density, which poses the danger of osteoporosis (loss of bone mass) in later years.

Be sure to consume enough foods that are rich in calcium, such as dairy products and salmon. You may want to take calcium supplements, even in a simple form (like an antacid), to make sure that your intake is adequate—but be sure to consult your physician before taking this step.

Performance-Enhancing Substances

Once the domain of professional and elite athletes, substances such as steroids and other legal and illegal performance enhancers have now trickled down to the college and high school level. Most of these substances are banned by professional leagues and sports governing bodies, and cautionary tales about their often dangerous side effects abound. Still, this has not stopped many younger athletes from experimenting with them in hopes of enhancing their athletic performance.

Steroids

Anabolic steroids, the synthetic derivatives of male hormones, have been shown to increase lean muscle mass; they are therefore often used by athletes in sports that require strength, such as football. They are also illegal, banned by virtually every professional and amateur athletic organization because of their dangerous side effects, which include liver damage, elevated blood pressure, mood swings and aggression, heart disease, and impaired immune function.

Since anabolic steroids increase the levels of testosterone in the blood, they can have the effect of causing masculine characteristics in women, such as increased muscularity, deepening of the voice, and increased facial hair.

Human Growth Hormone

Human growth hormone (HGH) is produced in the body by the pituitary gland and is thought to enhance performance when taken in higher concentrations, usually by injection. It is banned by the major international sports governing bodies, but it is believed to be widely used in some sports and is very difficult to detect. Increasing the level of HGH in the body is thought to increase protein retention and thereby provide a slight advantage in adding muscle. However, the advantage is minor compared to the potential side effects of taking too much HGH: excessive perspiration, hypertension (abnormally high blood pressure), diabetes, widening of the jaw, enlarged facial features, and arthritis.

Creatine and Androstenedione

Creatine, or creatine monohydrate, is an over-the-counter supplement in powder form that assists in the production of adenosine triphosphate in the muscles, enabling the muscles to work harder. It has been shown to help athletes gain more muscle, power, and mass, and is reportedly used by many professional athletes. However, many professional teams have banned its use because of reports of side effects such as headache, stomach cramps, elevated blood pressure, and severe muscle cramps.

Androstenedione (andro), a supplement taken in pill form, received a great deal of publicity in 1998 when it was discovered that baseball slugger Mark McGwire was taking it during his quest for the all-time single-season home run mark. Although classified as a dietary supplement, andro actually simulates anabolic steroids and has been claimed to increase the level of testosterone in the blood, thus aiding an increase in muscle development. However, a 1999 study published in the *Journal of the American Medical Association* found that it not only did not increase testosterone levels, but actually increased the levels of estrogen (a female hormone), in male subjects, as well as increased cholesterol levels in the blood.

Summary

Fortunately, along with the explosion of supplements and performance-enhancing substances on the market has come a corresponding wealth of literature detailing the potential dangers inherent in their use. Any athlete—at any level of experience or ability—should make himself or herself fully aware of the risks before even considering using any of these substances.

FITNESS AND WEIGHT LOSS

Many people embarking on a fitness program list losing weight as one of their primary goals, and there certainly is a direct correlation between "getting in shape" and losing weight. If you are exercising regularly but cannot seem to lose weight, relax—you may be healthier than you think. A study released in 2002 by the Cooper Institute of Dallas found that a moderate to high level of cardiorespiratory fitness reduced the risk of death in women with an average age of 43 by as much as 52 percent. The study concluded that cardiorespiratory fitness is a better predictor of mortality in women than body mass index (body weight multiplied by 703, then divided by height in inches).

This conclusion, by itself, could be the strongest argument for regular exercise. But it also highlights another important fact: In a culture obsessed with body image in which the ideal is a runway model (for women) and a bodybuilder (for men), being healthy is defined using different criteria.

The message here is that if you exercise regularly but do not see tangible results on your bathroom scale, this does not mean that your workouts are not effective. The problem may be related to your diet, for instance, and may mean you need to reduce your consumption of fatty foods. Or it may be related to your body type: Overweight people often are physically fit and have healthy blood pressure and cholesterol levels—if they exercise regularly and eat a balanced diet.

If you are succeeding in your goal to lose weight, remember that losing too much weight too fast is not healthy either. Rapid weight loss can cause you to lose muscle tissue in addition to fat.

There are limitations to what an overweight person should expect to be able to do, of course. It may be wise to avoid running, for instance, and opt instead for low-impact activities, like swimming and cycling, that build cardiorespiratory fitness. If you are overweight, nothing should stop you from combining these and other forms of exercise with a balanced diet.

12

Buying Home Fitness Equipment

Home fitness equipment can be a boon or a bane. If you buy the right equipment for your needs and goals, and you are sufficiently motivated to use it on a regular basis, the benefits can be enormous. Spreading out the cost of a home gym or treadmill or elliptical trainer over the course of a year can be cheaper than some gym memberships, and you can use it whenever and however you want.

On the other hand, if you buy a machine that winds up in the corner gathering dust, you will have wasted your money and not improved your fitness either. A look at the classified ads in your local newspaper under Merchandise for Sale will tell you what becomes of many treadmills, cross-country trainers, and rowing machines.

What is the solution? First, know what you are looking for, and once you've found it, get the best model you can afford. Of course, that is only half the battle. The other half is to realize that despite the claims of many TV hucksters who claim their products will give you a lean, muscular body in 10 minutes a day, it is going to take a solid commitment on your part to make it

happen. The right equipment can make losing weight and toning your body much easier. This chapter describes the basic types of home exercise units and gives tips on buying the right one for you.

MAKING SPACE

What kind of home exercise equipment you buy is dictated to a large degree by your living space. Fortunately, many modern exercise units are models of efficiency and can be folded up and stored in a closet or corner. Still, make sure that you have a room that is well lit and well ventilated and gives you enough space to move around without feeling claustrophobic. Many people find it helpful to set up their equipment in a room that has a television within viewing distance.

THE RIGHT MACHINE FOR YOU

There is a dizzying array of home fitness machines on the market today. It is good to have choices, but the sheer

147

number of machines makes the task of choosing the right one more complicated. There are treadmills and elliptical trainers, abdominal machines and exercise bikes, rowing machines and multistation home gyms that look like the ones at your local health club.

Since this is likely to be a big investment, it is worth taking the time to research the different types of machines, and then research the available brands when you have chosen the type you want.

First, decide what your goals are. Do you want to build your endurance and cardiorespiratory fitness? (A treadmill makes sense.) Do you want to increase your muscle size? (Free weights would do the trick.) Do you want to lose your love handles and develop a flatter stomach? (An abdominal machine would help, either as a separate piece of equipment or as part of a gym unit.) Do you want to do all of these things?

Do you have an injury or medical condition that would rule out some types of exercises? (Don't buy a rowing machine if you have lower back problems, and maybe not a treadmill; a nonimpact elliptical trainer might be best.)

Before the basic types of home exercise machines are described, it is important to know how you would use them. Here is some general advice on using home exercise equipment:

- Strive for balance in your workouts. Strength, flexibility, and aerobic capacity are the three essential components of fitness. If you run on a regular basis, you might want to consider buying free weights or a home gym unit to add strength training to your routine.
- If you have an injury or medical condition that would affect your workout, seek the advice of a physi-

cian or orthopedist before buying any exercise machine.
- An injury or medical condition usually does not mean that you have to curtail your training. In fact, physical activity is far preferable to inactivity when you are rehabilitating most injuries. People with injured or subpar knees can still ride a stationary bike, and people with lower back pain can still train effectively, provided they perform the correct stretching and strengthening exercises.
- Most exercise machines have features that allow you to increase the speed or intensity of the workout. Use the lower settings initially, and move up when you feel comfortable doing so. Assuming that you stick with your workout schedule, you will want to increase the intensity and duration of your workouts. To avoid injury, this should be done gradually.
- Despite claims by manufacturers, no machine can give you a total workout. Treadmills don't develop your upper body, and free weights don't increase your endurance. Don't rely on a single machine to be your only training tool.

Following is a description of the basic types of home exercise machines and the features to look for if you are thinking of buying one.

Treadmills

Treadmills are probably the biggest seller among types of home fitness equipment. They offer an ideal way to burn calories, increase cardiovascular capacity, and strengthen the lower body by allowing you to perform running and walking motions. They let you adjust your workout by changing speed, as well as the angle of incline (so that you are running or walking uphill). Perhaps most important, they offer cushioning to minimize stress on your joints—which is one of the big drawbacks of running outdoors on surfaces like asphalt and concrete.

Treadmills consist of a looped belt mounted on a sturdy deck and propelled by an electric motor, although some models have no motor and are propelled by your own power. Many have electronic features that allow you to preprogram varying levels of speed and incline during your workout. Some also keep track of how many calories you are burning (though one should be skeptical of this, since it depends on several factors, such as your body weight and your food intake before your workout).

Features to Look For

- A cushioned deck that absorbs shock but is firm (If you are overweight or have joint problems, you should look for a deck with more cushioning.)
- A deck that is at least 18 inches wide
- Variable speeds up to five or 10 mph (If you will only be walking on your treadmill, look for one with a maximum speed of 5 mph and a deck that is of average length. If you will be running on the treadmill, look for one that has speeds up to 10 mph (or even higher) and a longer deck to accommodate a longer stride.)
- Self-lubricating parts
- An electronic console that isn't confusing (The console should be easy to understand and easy to operate.)
- Controls that let you increase belt speed gradually, particularly when starting up
- Preset workout programs that are interesting and challenging
- A heart rate monitor (Some treadmill models use a chest strap to monitor your heart rate.)

- Safety features: a removable stop key, handrails, and a safety lock
- A one-year warranty on labor and one to three years on parts

Stair-Climbers

Stair-climbers provide an excellent workout for your calves, thighs, buttocks, hips, and lower back, with significantly less impact than jogging or running. However, they may exacerbate a preexisting knee problem, so it is important to consult with your physician or physical therapist before you buy one.

There are two types of stair-climbers: those that use dependent steps and those that use independent steps. Some machines combine both. Beginners are usually advised to use dependent steppers, since they are easier to use. As you push one step down, the other rises. Independent steppers are more complicated; they require you to work both feet at once. It may take some time to adjust to the motion of an independent stepper so that you don't lose your balance, but once you are accustomed to the motion, you get a more challenging workout.

Resistance, or the intensity of the workout, is adjusted manually or with computerized controls, depending on the type of machine. Stair-climbers with computerized controls are more expensive, but they make up for the extra cost in convenience. Some models have a feature that estimates how many calories you are burning.

Features to Look For

- A sturdy frame that doesn't tilt or wobble while you are using it
- Dependent or independent steps, or both
- A heart rate monitor
- A variety of preset programs, plus the ability to create your own custom program

- Low noise (Machines that use hydraulic pistons are often louder.)

Elliptical Trainers

These low-impact machines are a cross between a stair-climber and a cross-country ski machine. They simulate a natural way of moving, which makes them easy for beginners to use right away, and they are great for athletes who have suffered bone and joint injuries. Early elliptical trainers focused solely on foot motion, which provided only a lower body workout. Current machines feature arm handles, so that the upper body and lower body are worked together. Simultaneous working of the upper and lower body can increase muscle tone and provide a more powerful cardiovascular stimulus than if you worked the two areas separately.

Probably the most important feature of the elliptical trainer is that it provides a low-impact workout. Your feet do not leave the footpads, which is essential for people with problem joints that can't withstand a lot of pounding. Since there is little wasted motion when you use an elliptical trainer, the workout is very efficient. In addition, the machine stops when you do, which is an important safety point.

Features to Look For

- A sturdy frame that doesn't wobble or tilt and hand grips that are comfortable and secure
- An elliptical motion so that your heel does not come off the footpad (The motion should feel smooth throughout; you shouldn't feel a "kick.")
- Comfortable motions that are not awkward (for ellipticals that offer upper and lower body resistance) (This is especially important if you have a preexisting joint problem.)

- An adjustable incline and adjustable resistance (These features can add challenge to your workout and vary the focus on different muscle groups. Adjusting the resistance can add an interval training component to your workout.)
- Forward and reverse motions (This can add variety to your workout and reduce your risk of developing repetitive stress injuries.)
- An electronic console that is useful and easy to understand and includes features like the number of calories you are burning
- Preset programs that are challenging and motivating
- A warranty that covers electronics

Cross-Country Ski Machines

Cross-country skiing is generally considered to be one of the best, most efficient forms of aerobic exercise because it offers a total body workout with very low impact. While cross-country ski machines are much easier to use than learning to ski in the snow, they do require you to develop balance and coordination. It will probably take you some time to get used to moving your arms and legs in different rhythms. Don't rush it.

Cross-country ski machines use long, narrow boards or footpads in place of skis, and these glide on rollers. A rope or pulley system simulates the motion of ski poles. The skis themselves can be dependent or independent, and the difference is a crucial one. Dependent skis are linked, so that when one moves forward, the other moves back. These machines are good for beginners who need to get used to the skiing motion, but they offer no variation—you are forced to follow the machine's cadence.

Machines that use independent ski motion rely on you to move each ski separately, which is a more natural motion and better simulates actual cross-country skiing. Independent ski motion also provides a more intense workout than dependent, but it can be harder for beginners to master.

Features to Look For

- Dependent or independent ski motion (This is the most basic decision you need to make before buying. Try out both types to determine your ability level and which type is right for you.)
- A smooth motion that allows you to make comfortable strides and arm movements that aren't tight or jerky (This can only be discovered if you try before you buy.)
- A long platform on which the skis slide back and forth (Many health club models have this feature, while many home models use boards that resemble skis. The platform can feel more stable and provide a somewhat bigger comfort zone for beginners.)
- A computerized control pad that displays distance traveled, time, and speed (Some models also monitor your heart rate and the number of calories you are burning.)
- Programmable resistance settings (These can simulate different snow types, as well as changing terrain. Uphill skiing provides a more vigorous workout for your front thigh muscles.)
- Vinyl hip support pads, available on some models
- The ability to be folded up for easy storage
- A warranty of at least one year on parts and labor

Stationary Bicycles

If you love cycling but are unable to ride outside—for example, if you live in the northeastern United States from November through February—a stationary bicycle can be a savior, both physically and psychologically. You get a nonimpact workout, and you control the pace and intensity. A stationary bicycle is recommended for people who are overweight or have joint problems.

There are several types of stationary bicycles. The first is, believe it or not, your own bike. You can attach your back wheel to a device called a wind trainer, which employs a roller that can be adjusted to provide different degrees of resistance. The advantages of the wind trainer are that you are using a bike you already feel comfortable riding, and that you can shift gears as you would if you were riding on the road to change speed or intensity.

A basic stationary bike lets you set the resistance manually. Computerized models regulate the resistance electronically and let you program different workouts. Many bikes also have movable handlebars that can be pumped back and forth to give you an upper body workout.

A relatively recent trend in cycling is the use of recumbent bikes. Built with the pedals in front of you, these bikes are operated with your legs extended forward and your upper body leaning back instead of in an upright position. This is a significant breakthrough in exercise technology, because it takes strain off your lower back and focuses on your leg muscles: the hamstrings and quads.

Features to Look For

- Features that fit your exercise goals and your physical requirements (For instance, do you want a bike with movable handlebars for an upper body workout?)
- A stable unit that doesn't tilt or wobble (A bike with a heavier front wheel will usually be more stable.)
- A comfortable, easily adjusted seat
- Adjustable handlebars

- Computerized controls that are easy to read and within easy reach
- Preset programs, as well as the ability to create custom programs
- Holders for a water bottle, reading material, or portable music player

Rowing Machines

Rowing machines offer a great total body workout, but with a huge disclaimer: If you have any kind of back problem, proceed with caution. In fact, it might be wise to avoid this type of exercise altogether. Even athletes with healthy backs can strain muscles from rowing. However, rowing strengthens your arms, legs, shoulders, and back with very low impact. It can also hook you—ask any dedicated rower. You may eventually find yourself out on a lake in a real boat.

The water (and air, to a degree) provides resistance when you are rowing on a lake. In the gym or at home, rowing machines rely on different types of resistance. Standard rowing machines use air resistance generated by a flywheel, which has a smooth, steady motion. Other models use a water flywheel, which more closely approximates real rowing. Still others use pistons or cylinders.

Features to Look For

- A comfortable, adjustable seat and footpads
- A bar or handles that are comfortable and easy to grip
- A fitness monitor that tracks time, speed, and distance and estimates the number of calories you are burning
- The ability to stand on end or be folded for easy storage
- Low noise (Models that use a flywheel tend to be louder, but some flywheel models are quieter than others.)

Free Weights

Free weights are one of the basic building blocks of a home gym;

you can add pieces over time without spending a large sum of money up front. Training with free weights is quite different from using a weight machine, and it requires considerably more practice and technique to avoid injury. The leading cause of injuries involving weights is incorrect technique. For this reason, it is often best for beginners to use weight machines that restrict range of motion with weights. If you wish to start out with free weights, be absolutely sure to seek instruction on technique and safety from trained professionals.

If you are using barbells, it is recommended that you have a partner to act as a spotter. If you are lifting alone, dumbbells are a safer alternative and can provide a similar workout.

With dumbbells, start out with at least four or five pairs, ranging in weight from 2.5 to as much as 45 pounds, depending on how much you normally lift (or realistically see yourself lifting in the future). Buy larger dumbbells in five- to 10-pound increments.

Barbells come in different weights and shapes. Hex bars are shaped like a hexagon with handles for doing shrugs and dead lifts, and curl bars have dips in the middle. Whatever weight or shape your barbell is, you will need weight plates to put on it. Start out with four each of the 10-, 5-, and 2.5-pound sizes.

For dumbbells and (especially) barbells, you also need a weight bench. There is a wide variety to consider, from basic flat benches that rest on two legs, to flat benches with adjustable legs (they resemble an ironing board), to incline benches, to adjustable benches that feature racks that hold weights and attachments for leg exercises.

Features to Look For

- Hexagonal heads on dumbbells (so they don't roll on the floor)

(This applies to weight plates too; any shape but round is fine.)

- Comfortable hand grips on barbells and dumbbells
- Locking collars for weight plates that are secure but don't gouge the plates
- A sturdy weight bench made of heavy-duty commercial steel
- An adjustable weight bench (adjustable to *your* measurements)

Multistation Gyms

Multistation home gyms have become tremendously popular in recent years, and it is easy to see why. They offer most, if not all, of the exercises you can perform in a gym. One standard model, for instance, lets you do chin-ups and dips, pec flyes, lat pulldowns, low rows, leg extensions and leg curls, preacher curls and bench presses, squats, shrugs, and more. Another advantage is that the machine takes up relatively little space.

A home gym uses one of three types of resistance:

- Weight stacks. You insert a pin into the stack to select how much weight you want to lift. The stack is then lifted via a cable or pulley system. Not surprisingly, these machines are the least portable, but they may be the sturdiest. They also make it easy to change weights.
- Hydraulic pistons. These machines rely on fluid in cylinders being forced from one chamber to another. You adjust the resistance by using valves or by changing the point at which a piston is attached to levers. There is no resistance on the eccentric, or return, part of a motion (that is, when you are bringing the weight back down).
- Flexible rods and rubber bands. These are attached to the frame and to the cable you are moving. These machines tend to be lightweight and

are more portable than the other two types.

Since these machines are more complex than any other type of equipment you are likely to purchase, you should spend time testing different models. First, consider your fitness goals, as well as the goals of anyone else who would be using the equipment. Weight machines force you to follow a specific motion with each exercise, and depending on your height and weight, that motion may not suit your body type. This makes it even more imperative to try out a machine by performing all your exercises on it.

As a general rule, it is usually best not to "underbuy"—that is, don't buy something you may outgrow in the near future. Look for a home gym that has a wide range of settings and enough weight or resistance so that you won't find yourself outperforming the machine. Also, make sure that your available space at home has enough square footage so that you can move freely around the unit as you go from one exercise to the next.

Finally, the adage about getting what you pay for holds especially true here. With such a wide variety of machines available in a wide price range, spending a few extra dollars up front can make a significant difference later.

Features to Look For

- A unit that fits your body type and allows a full range of motion during each exercise
- A smooth, quiet motion (Some types of pulleys are quieter than others. This is one of the reasons why you should try out several machines.)
- A sturdy frame constructed of 11-gauge steel, with a paint finish that repels moisture and resists corrosion (The unit must feel stable and capable of withstanding continuous stress; it needs to be strongest

at welded joints (somewhat like the joints of your body).)

- Pads of molded polyurethane, which won't crack or peel with use (and won't smell, either)
- Adjustability (This enables you to always be in the correct position to do the exercise correctly.)
- Ease of setup for different exercises (This enables you to move quickly from one exercise to the next, which is the key to circuit training.)
- Portability (If you have space restrictions and will need to move the unit regularly, you probably shouldn't buy a unit with weight stacks.)
- Ease of assembly (Larger, heavier machines may be more difficult to put together.)
- A wall chart that describes and illustrates all the exercises and an instructional video (Watch the video—you will pick up pointers about getting the maximum benefit from the machine.)
- Adaptability (This enables you to add accessories to the basic machine.)
- A warranty that covers the frame, cables, and upholstery (The machine should come with an extended warranty, so that you don't have to pay extra for an extension.)

Abdominal Machines

With so many products on the market offering miracle cures for flabby stomachs, it is easy to dismiss all the claims as so much hot air. The truth is, however, that many of these machines can actually help tone and tighten your abdominal muscles. The key is to find one that is dependable, easy to use, and not hazardous to your lower back.

Abdominal machines come in several basic models. They use rollers, sliders, wheels, and/or belts. Some units consist of a board with footpads that can be placed flat or on an incline. Other units use arm resistance to simu-

late the crunch motion from a seated position. Some units feature a separate chin-up and dip station for knee raises and other abdominal exercises.

If you are only concerned with working on your abs and you have limited space, a unit with rollers and sliders may be best; such units are lightweight and can fold up or be stored in a closet. If you want a more total body workout, you should consider a home gym that features apparatus for abdominal exercises.

Features to Look For

- Lower back support (This feature is critical and may be the most important consideration. Of course, proper technique is also important, but that is your responsibility.)
- Sturdy construction
- A design that is suited to your body type and makes the unit comfortable to use
- Adaptability (This enables you to add weight or resistance to the exercise(s).)

Exercise Balls (Swiss Balls)

Originally used in Switzerland to help people with orthopedic injuries, these balls are now used all over the world by athletes and nonathletes who want to develop their coordination and balance. They also provide an alternative method of performing some traditional exercises like push-ups and squats and are used in core strengthening programs that focus on developing the muscles of the trunk. There are dozens of exercises that can be done using exercise balls, each targeting a specific muscle group.

If you choose to train with an exercise ball, keep in mind that balance will be of paramount importance. The ball's pliancy forces you to use the muscles of your lower back, trunk, and pelvis continuously to maintain balance during exercises. For instance, performing crunches while balancing your back on the balance ball forces you to focus on the exercise as well as on keeping your back in position so that you don't fall off.

Features to Look For

- Balls that are proportionate to your height and to the exercises you will be performing (Sizes range from small (22 inches in diameter) for people 5'0" to 5'5", medium (26 inches) for people 5'5" to 5'11", and large (30 inches) for people 6'0" foot and above.)
- Construction of soft PVC material that can withstand heavy weights (If you are overweight, check the maximum weight the ball can handle.)
- A video or pamphlet that describes and illustrates exercises that you can perform (You should actually get this information from your trainer or physical therapist, since proper technique is absolutely essential when using a balance ball.)

TIPS ON BUYING HOME FITNESS EQUIPMENT

Buying home fitness equipment involves a large investment of money at the beginning, and using it involves a large investment of time thereafter.

If you make the right choice, your investment will pay off on both ends. Here are general guidelines to follow when buying exercise equipment for use in your home:

- Purchase equipment only if you are going to commit yourself to using it at least two or three times per week. The most expensive, high-tech machine in the world won't do you any good if you only use it to hang laundry on.
- Wear workout clothes to the store and test the equipment as you will really use it. See how your body feels later in the day and on the day after testing the equipment.
- If exercise feels awkward or uncomfortable while you are testing the equipment, reconsider your reasons for wanting to buy it.
- You cannot break in equipment. If it feels uncomfortable during testing in the store, it will feel uncomfortable when it is in your home.
- Some dealers may allow you to take a machine home to test it. Take advantage of this option, if available, and don't feel shy about sending it back.
- Certain machines fit individual body types better. If you find equipment you like at a health club, find a dealer who sells it.

GLOSSARY

Abdominal muscles The muscles that lie between the thorax and pelvis: the rectus abdominis and the external obliques.

Abduction Movement of a limb away from the middle of the body. When performing hip abduction exercises, a person starts with the legs together and moves one or both outward.

Adduction Movement of a limb toward the middle of the body. When performing hip adduction exercises, a person starts with the legs apart and moves one or both inward.

Aerobic exercise/training Training designed to improve the body's circulatory and respiratory efficiency through sustained, vigorous exercise. Jogging is an example of an aerobic exercise.

Anaerobic exercise/training Training that focuses on short, explosive actions. Sprinting is an example of an anaerobic exercise.

Androstenedione A performance-enhancing supplement that has been claimed to have effects similar to those of anabolic steroids, for example, increasing the level of testosterone in the blood.

Barbell A metal bar used in weight lifting, five to seven feet long, with detachable weights at each end.

Biaxial joint A joint that allows two types of movement in two directions. The wrist and ankle are biaxial joints.

Biceps The muscle at the front of the upper arm that flexes the forearm.

Blood-sugar level The concentration of glucose in the blood, measured in milligrams of glucose per 100 milliliters of blood.

Calcium An element found in compound form in dairy and other products that contributes to healthy bones and teeth. A calcium deficiency can lead to osteoporosis (decreased bone mass).

Calorie A unit of energy-producing potential that is contained in food and released upon oxidation by the body.

Carbohydrate An organic compound that, when broken down by the body, becomes glucose molecules that the body can use for energy. Simple carbohydrates include refined and naturally occurring sugars. Complex carbohydrates are found in breads, pasta, fruits, and vegetables.

Cardiovascular exercise Exercise that raises the heart rate and gets blood flowing to the muscles and joints.

Concentric action The shortening of a muscle that occurs when weight is lifted.

Cooldown A post-workout routine that lets the body make the transition from being stressed to being at rest. This helps the muscles remove some of the lactic acid buildup after a strenuous workout.

Creatine An over-the-counter supplement that assists in the production of adenosine triphosphate in the muscles, enabling them to work harder. It has been banned by many sports governing bodies.

Cross-training Training that combines aerobic, anaerobic, and resistance exercises.

Detraining The decrease in strength and conditioning that occurs when a training program is suspended.

Dietary/nutritional supplement A mineral, amino acid, or other substance claimed to improve athletic performance, but not claimed to have any specific therapeutic value and thus not regulated by the Food and Drug Administration (FDA).

Dumbbell A metal bar used in weight lifting, about 14 inches long, with detachable or fixed weights at each end. It is used, usually in pairs, in hand exercises such as wrist curls and biceps curls.

Dynamic muscle action A resistance exercise that involves motion, such as when a weight is raised (concentric action) and then lowered (eccentric action).

Eccentric action The lengthening of a muscle that occurs during deceleration, such as when a weight is lowered to its starting position.

Elastic resistance A system of springs or rubber bands used in many home gym units. These machines provide low resistance at the beginning of a motion and high resistance toward the end.

Extension Movement of a limb or joint from a bent to a straight position.

Fast-twitch muscle fibers Muscle fibers that develop force quickly over a short period of time. They are used in anaerobic exercises, such as sprinting.

Flexion Movement of a limb or joint from a straight to a bent position.

Fluid resistance The type of resistance employed in exercise machines that use cylinders and pistons rather than traditional weights.

Free weights Dumbbells, barbells, and plates that are freestanding and not attached to pulleys, pistons, or other apparatus. They allow more range of motion than weight machines, but require more focus on technique and balance.

Friction resistance The type of resistance employed in some exercise machines, such as some cycling machines.

Glucose A blood sugar that is the major source of energy for the body.

Glycemic index A system that measures how quickly a food is converted to glucose in the bloodstream.

Hamstring The three muscles (semitendinosus, semimembranosus, and biceps femoris) that run along the back of the thigh and behind the knee. They are used to flex the knee and extend the thigh.

Hormone A substance produced in the body that regulates physiological activity, such as growth or metabolism.

Human growth hormone A hormone produced in the body by the pituitary gland that is thought to enhance performance when taken in high concentrations, usually by injection. It is banned by the major international sports governing bodies.

Hypertrophy An increase in muscle size.

Intensity The percentage of one's repetition maximum (RM) used during an exercise or workout.

Isolation (of muscles) Focusing on a specific muscle or muscle group and performing exercises to overload it.

Isometric muscle action Muscle contraction where muscle length does not change and joints do not move. This occurs in exercises that involve pushing against an immovable object.

Lactic acid An organic acid produced by intense anaerobic activity that builds up in muscles and causes fatigue.

Latissimus dorsi muscles (lats) The large muscles of the back that extend from just below the shoulder blades to the sides.

Ligament A band of tissue that connects bones or supports an organ.

Medicine ball A large, heavy ball, usually bound in leather and used in conditioning exercises.

Mineral An essential nutritional compound, such as calcium, iron, potassium, and sodium, that helps regulate many of the body's functions.

Motor nerve/neuron A neuron that conveys impulses from the central nervous system to muscles.

Motor unit The combination of a motor neuron and the muscle fibers to which it is attached.

Multiaxial joint A joint that allows movement in three directions. The shoulder, hip, and knee are multiaxial joints.

Multiple-joint exercise An exercise that involves movement at more than one joint. Examples are back squats and deadlifts.

Muscle endurance The ability of a muscle or muscle group to contract repeatedly for an extended period of time, such as during sit-ups.

Muscle fiber The cells that make up muscles. These long, cylindrical cells, about the diameter of a human hair, are grouped in bundles of up to 150, called fasciculi.

Muscle group A group of muscles that combine to perform a particular function. For example, the quadriceps (front thigh muscles) is a muscle group made up of four muscles: the rectus femoris, vastus lateralis, vastus medialis, and vastus intermedius. This muscle group flexes the hip and extends the knee.

Muscle imbalance Strengthening some muscle groups at the expense of others, such as by performing only one type of activity or sport.

Nutrient A source of nourishment found in food.

Overloading The act of forcing a muscle to do more than it is used to doing, enabling it to increase in size and strength.

Overtraining A condition unique to athletes in which excessive training causes fatigue, mood swings, depression, and altered sleeping and eating habits.

Performance-enhancing supplement A substance used specifically to improve or enhance performance.

Periodization A system of training that varies workout intensity and alternates exercises over a period of weeks or months.

Phosphagen An energy-supplying chemical composed of creatine and phosphate produced during the breakdown of adenosine triphosphate during anaerobic activity. Phosphagens are thought to support high-intensity anaerobic activity for about six to 10 seconds.

Power The rate of force (force times speed), or how fast a person is able to move an object.

Protein A naturally occurring compound composed of amino acids, obtained from many dietary sources, especially meat, eggs, and dairy products. Protein helps build muscles, blood, and organs, as well as assists in the formation of hormones, enzymes, and antibodies.

Quadriceps The group of four muscles in the front of the thigh that attach to the quadriceps tendon, which attaches to the kneecap. When the quadriceps muscles are flexed, the quadriceps tendon pulls on the kneecap and straightens the leg.

Range of motion The normal movement of a joint. Regaining range of motion is one of the first steps in rehabilitating an injury.

Recovery The period between exercises or workouts during which the body adapts to the stresses imposed by resistance training.

Repetition A single complete movement of an exercise, from the starting position, through the movement, back to the starting position. The number of repetitions ("reps") is the number of times an exercise is performed during one set.

Repetition maximum (RM) The maximum weight that a person can lift for a specific number of repetitions to exhaustion. For example, if a person can bench press 100 pounds 10 times but no more, his or her 10RM for the bench press is 100 pounds.

Resistance training Training that requires the exertion of force against a movable or immovable object.

Rest period The time between sets or exercises in a workout, usually between 30 seconds and three or four minutes.

RICE An acronym that stands for **R**est, **I**ce, **C**ompression, and **E**levation. It is the best and easiest method for treating minor muscle injuries, such as pulls and strains.

Rotator cuff A group of four muscles originating at the shoulder blade and forming one continuous cuff across the shoulder. It controls the rotation of the ball-shaped head of the upper arm bone in the shoulder socket, keeping the ball centered in the socket as it rotates.

Set A group of repetitions of a specific exercise, followed by a short rest period.

Single-joint exercise An exercise that involves movement at only one joint, usually to train a single muscle or muscle group. Examples are arm curls and knee extensions.

Slow-twitch muscle fibers Muscle fibers that develop force slowly over a long period of time. They provide energy and endurance during aerobic activities.

Specificity Tailoring a training program to a specific activity or sport by adding, subtracting, or altering exercises.

Sports drink A specially manufactured drink that contains extra carbohydrates.

Spotter A person who assists a weight lifter during an exercise, particularly if the exercise involves heavy weights or is technically difficult.

Steroid, anabolic A synthetic derivative of male hormones that increases the level of testosterone in the blood. In women, it may cause the development of masculine characteristics, such as increased muscularity, deepening of the voice, and increased facial hair. Anabolic steroids are banned by college and professional sports organizations and the Olympics.

Strength The ability of a muscle to exert maximum force.

Stretching Exercises designed to loosen up muscles, ligaments, and joints in preparation for a workout. Stretching helps prevent injury.

Target heart rate (THR) The rate at which the heart should be pumping during exercise to get the maximum cardiovascular benefit. The THR is a percentage of the maximum heart rate and varies from person to person, depending on age and fitness level.

Tendinitis Inflammation of a tendon or tendons as a result of overuse of a particular joint. Tendinitis in athletes is common in the knees, shoulders, and elbows.

Tendon A band of fibrous tissue that connects a muscle to a bone.

Testosterone A steroid hormone produced by the body that is responsible for the development and maintenance of male secondary sex characteristics.

Triceps The large muscle at the back of the upper arm that extends the forearm.

Uniaxial joint A joint that allows movement in only one direction, like a hinge. The elbow is a uniaxial joint.

Universal machine A type of exercise machine that features weights on tracks or rails being lifted by pulleys or levers.

Visualization A technique used to vividly imagine the activity a person is about to perform, so that the brain and nervous system are better prepared to put the thought into action.

Vitamin An organic compound derived from plants and animals that is essential for the body's growth and maintenance.

Warm-up A series of light exercises or stretching that serves to increase blood flow to the muscles before a workout or competition.

Weightlifting belt A wide belt, made of leather or a synthetic material, worn by weight lifters to support the lower back during lifting.

Weight machine An exercise machine that uses weights to provide resistance. It requires less focus on technique and balance and is generally easier to use than free weights.

INDEX

Certain exercises are designated as part of a training program or workout.

AT Alternative training   WB Women's beginner
MB Men's beginner   WI Women's intermediate
MI Men's intermediate

THE STORY OF GOLD'S GYM

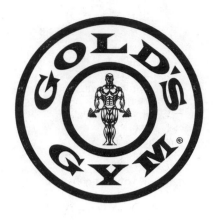

Gold's Gym has been the authority on fitness since 1965 dating back to the original Gold's Gym in Venice, California. It was the place for serious fitness. Gold's Gym quickly became known as "The Mecca of Bodybuilding." In 1977, Gold's Gym received international attention when it was featured in the movie *Pumping Iron* that starred Arnold Schwarzenegger and Lou Ferrigno. From that first gym in Venice, Gold's Gym has become the largest co-ed gym chain in the world with over 550 facilities in 43 states and 25 countries.

Today, Gold's Gym has expanded its fitness profile to offer all of the latest equipment and services, including group exercise, personal training, cardiovascular equipment, group spin, pilates and yoga, while maintaining its core weight lifting tradition. With nearly 3 million members world wide, Gold's Gym continues to change lives by helping people achieve their individual potential. For more information about Gold's Gym, please visit www.goldsgym.com or call 1-800-99-GOLDS.

Gold's Gym has the classes you want, the equipment you need and the trainers to help you get the results you're looking for!

The Latest Equipment • Certified Personal Training • Nutrition Counseling • Extensive Cardio • Women's Only Areas • Childcare
Plus Hundreds of Group Exercise Classes including: Group Spin • Yoga • Pilates • Kickboxing • Step • Stretch and More!

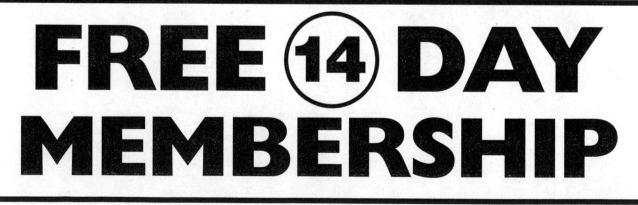

FREE (14) DAY MEMBERSHIP

First time visitors only. Must be over 18 with valid ID. Must be local resident. Not redeemable for cash. Participating Gold's Gyms only. Other restrictions may apply. Amenities vary by location. ©2004 Gold's Gym International, Inc.

Log on to www.goldsgym.com/bookoffer
or call 1-800-99-GOLDS
to get your free pass today!